New Careers In Nursing

New Careers In Nursing

Florence Downs, R.N., Ed.D., F.A.A.N.
Associate Dean and Director of Graduate Studies
University of Pennsylvania
School of Nursing

and

Dorothy Brooten, M.S.N., Ph.D., F.A.A.N.
Assistant Professor
University of Pennsylvania
School of Nursing

ARCO PUBLISHING, INC.
NEW YORK

Published by Arco Publishing, Inc.
215 Park Avenue South, New York, N.Y. 10003

Copyright © 1983 by Florence S. Downs and Dorothy A. Brooten

All rights reserved. No part of this book may be reproduced, by any means, without permission in writing from the publisher, except by a reviewer who wishes to quote brief excerpts in connection with a review in a magazine or newspaper.

Library of Congress Cataloging in Publication Data

Downs, Florence S.
  New careers in nursing.

  Includes index.
  1. Nursing—Vocational guidance. I. Brooten, Dorothy A. II. Title. [DNLM: 1. Specialties, Nursing. WY 101 D751w]
  RT82.D68   1983   610.73′06′9   82-18449
  ISBN 0-668-05255-4 (Reference Text)
  ISBN 0-668-05260-0 (pbk.)

Printed in the United States of America

Contents

Acknowledgments viii
Preface ix
1. Introduction to Nursing and Nursing Education 1

    Practical Nursing Programs 3
    Educational Preparation of Registered Nurses 3
        Diploma Programs 4
        Associate Degree Programs 5
        Baccalaureate Degree Programs 6
        Master's Degree Programs 8
        Doctoral Nursing Programs 10
    Choosing a Nursing Program 11
    Financing Your Education 13
    How to Get Started 14
    For Further Information 16

2. Hospitals 19

    Staff Nursing 20
        On a Surgical Unit 20
        Operating Room 22
        Emergency Room 27
        Surgical Intensive Care Unit 29
        Psychiatric Unit 32
        Labor and Delivery Unit 34
        Newborn Intensive Care Unit 37
        Newborn Transport Nursing 39
        Outpatient Clinic 40
        Other Staff Nursing Positions 43
    Types of Nursing Care Delivery 48
        Primary Nursing 48
        Team Nursing 48
        Functional Nursing 49
    In-Service Educator 49
    Clinical Specialist 52
    Head Nurse 56
    Assistant Director 60

  Director of Nursing or Chief Nurse Executive 62
  For Further Information 63

3. Independent and Joint Practices 66

  Adult Nurse Clinician 68
  Family Nurse Clinician 69
  Certified Nurse Midwife 70
  Pediatric Nurse Clinician 73
  Psychiatric Nurse Practitioner 74
  Neonatal Nurse Practitioner 75
  Certified Registered Nurse Anesthetist (CRNA) 76
  Nurse Practitioner in a College Health Service 77
  For Further Information 79

4. Community Health 81

  School Nursing 85
  School Nursing for Emotionally Disturbed Children 86
  Camp Nursing 87
  Rural Nursing 91
  Occupational Health Nursing 92
  Occupational Health Nursing at Three Mile Island (TMI) 94
  For Further Information 97

5. Extended Care Facilities 100

  Nursing Homes 100
  Geriatric Nurse Practitioner 101
  Gerontological Nurse Specialist 102
  Rehabilitation Centers 104
  Nursing Developmentally Disabled Children 106
  Hospice Care 108
  For Further Information 110

6. Government Service 112

  Public Health Service 112
  Health Agencies of the U.S. Public Health Service 114
  Indian Health Service 115
  Locations for Nursing Positions in the Indian Health Service 118
  Nursing in the Armed Services 121
   Qualifications 121
   Orientation 122

      Nursing Assignments 122
      Army School Nurse 126
  Civil Service 126
  Veterans Administration 127
  Peace Corps and VISTA 130
  Nursing During War—One Nurse's Experience 130
  For Further Information 132

7. Education, Research, and Combined Careers 134

  Nurse Educators 134
    Practical Nursing Education 134
    Diploma Nursing Education 136
    Collegiate Programs 138
    Associate Degree Nursing Education 138
    Baccalaureate Degree Nursing Education 140
    Master's Degree Nursing Education 143
    Doctoral Degree Nursing Education 144
  Educational Administration 146
  Nursing Research 147
    Conducting Research 149
  Combined Careers 152
    The Nurse Editor 153
    International Consultation 154
    Nursing School Recruiter 155
    Combined Teaching and Practice Positions 155
  For Further Information 156

Appendix I.   Regional and State Offices of the National League for
               Nursing and the American Nurses Association 159
Appendix II. State Boards of Nursing 163
Appendix III. Nursing Journals and Publications 168
Index 177

Acknowledgments

Photographs are courtesy of the University of Pennsylvania, the Pennsylvania Nurses Association, the Visiting Nurse Society of Philadelphia, the U.S. Public Health Service, the Peace Corps, the Veterans Administration, and the Department of Defense.

Preface

During the past thirty years, dramatic changes have taken place in the health care delivery system. New knowledge and complex technologies have reshaped nursing practice, opening up new roles and opportunities. Nursing has become a challenging profession for men and women who want to choose from a variety of roles, not only in direct patient care but in administration, teaching, research or a combination of these. Schools, nursing homes, rural and urban clinics, hospices, health maintenance operations and businesses are among the places clamoring for highly qualified nurses. Many of the positions available offer a high degree of autonomy and excellent chances for career advancement.

Because these changes have come about so quickly, many people are not aware of them. Therefore, this book is not only written for those who are thinking about entering a career in nursing, but also for counselors and nurses who are thinking about a change but are unsure of the opportunities available. The major purpose of the book is to introduce the reader to the broad spectrum of satisfying possibilities in the new world of nursing.

New Careers In Nursing

1.

Introduction to Nursing and Nursing Education

Until this century, most people were nursed in their homes. Hospitals cared primarily for the very poor and the homeless. But little by little all this changed and the principal setting for patient care and nursing practice became the hospital. This trend is now being reversed due to increased emphasis on prevention and cost containment. Many hospital inpatient units are becoming smaller, others are consolidating and some are closing. Patients who remain in the hospital are more acutely ill and require care in highly specialized units. At the same time, patients are being discharged from hospitals earlier and need more skilled nursing care in their homes. Statistics published recently in the *American Journal of Nursing* indicate that in the five years from 1972 through 1977, the number of nurses employed in community settings almost doubled. The trend is projected to increase sharply in the decades ahead. Change is the key word in the nursing profession and the entire system of health care. Today, the functions and frontiers of nursing practice have expanded so greatly that it seems difficult to think of a place where people live where nurses do not touch them in some way. For you, as a nurse, this spells more opportunity, challenge and responsibility than ever before.

Nurses may practice in the traditional hospital or clinic, visit patients in their homes or care for them in storefronts, clinics, or mobile health vans. Ships and transport aircraft are health care facilities used by the armed services all over the world. Nurses are in Third World native villages with the Peace Corps and on American Indian reservations with the U.S. Public Health Service. They are even found in such unconventional settings as cocktail lounges and on street corners doing counseling and casefinding for alcohol abuse or venereal disease programs. Nurses practice as salaried professionals, or as independent practitioners charging a fee for service. Sometimes they are in partnership with one or more nurse practitioners or physicians, for a salary or for a percentage of the receipts of the practice. The settings for modern nursing practice are almost infinite because the services are varied and expanding rapidly in scope. The groups served are as diverse as the hundreds of thousands of actively practicing nurses themselves.

As the settings in which nurses practice have changed, educational preparation has likewise changed and expanded. Each major societal trend of the last generation has had its impact on nursing. The tremendous increase in new knowledge; the increased use of new technology; the rapid communication and dispersal of knowledge, and a far better informed and educated public is increasingly demanding a more humane system of health care delivery. The cumulative effect has been greater demands upon nurses to respond appropriately and professionally to these new and challenging situations. Knowledge and skills once thought to be needed by only a few nursing leaders are essential tools for each new nurse today. From traditional hospital-based education, preparation of nurses has moved increasingly into institutions of higher education, transforming nursing's apprenticeship approach into one of disciplined scholarship.

For nurses to be effective in practice today, no matter the setting, a broad-based general education is a requirement for preparation. Providing care to patients requires a knowledge of our society, its institutions and its entire system of health care delivery. Contemporary nurses need an understanding of the behavior of patients, what causes them to seek or refuse health care, and what will motivate them to change habits or lifestyles so they can improve their health. This in turn requires an understanding of—and sensitivity to—ethnic and cultural differences. A seemingly innocent pat on the head can evoke terror in the parents of an East Asian child. In their culture this gesture is taboo, since it is believed to remove the spirit from the child's body. It is that easy to turn an innocent gesture into a very negative encounter.

Professional nursing education builds on a broad educational base as a framework for teaching traditional technical skills and the newer skills of physical examination. There is renewed emphasis on caring for those already ill, and on health counseling, health education and health maintenance. Nursing students have experiences in many different health care settings and with models of nursing that emphasize flexibility in meeting the needs of patients. The professional educational component particularly emphasizes the need for the continued learning required of all professionals. In addition, nursing research has become a vital part of nursing education, providing nurses with the tools to understand the basic nature of nursing care, and its impact on patterns of care. Graduates of beginning programs in nursing have the opportunity to expand their functions and responsibilities by pursuing additional education on the master's and doctoral levels—educational preparation for leadership positions and practice in expanded roles.

Practical Nursing Programs

Programs to train practical nurses have existed since the late 1800s. Today, educational programs to prepare practical nurses are approximately one year in length and include a few basic science courses as well as nursing courses. Programs for practical nurses are often based in hospitals, private vocational schools and some public high schools. Tuitions and fees range from very little cost in public high schools to costs equal to or surpassing those of one year's tuition at a state college. Upon completion of the educational program, the graduate is eligible to take the state examination for licensed practical nurse (LPN).

After passing the examination, the LPN may work in any position requiring an LPN license. While many LPNs work in hospitals, many others care for patients with less acute illnesses, convalescent patients and patients with chronic diseases in their homes. LPNs work under the direction of a licensed physician or a registered nurse. Salaries for LPNs are lower than those for registered nurses and there are fewer opportunities for jobs and career advancement. To advance their careers, many LPNs pursue further education to become registered nurses. In recent years, admissions to practical nursing programs have been declining, although most recent figures indicate the number of admissions to these programs may have reached a plateau.

Educational Preparation of Registered Nurses

Graduates of several types of educational programs in nursing may take the state board examination to qualify for licensure as a registered nurse (see Figure 1, page 5). These types include diploma, associate degree and baccalaureate degree programs in nursing. They differ from each other in length and focus.

Since 1965, the American Nurses Association has taken the position that the baccalaureate degree should be the entry-level requirement of registered nurse licensure. Subsequently, many other nursing groups have come out in support of that position and job requirements increasingly reflect this stance. In February 1982, the Board of Directors of the National League for Nursing approved a position statement on the scope and preparation of nursing roles. The statement reads in part, "Given the need for such a broad background in the arts and sciences, as well as in nursing, professional nursing practice requires the minimum of a baccalaureate degree with a major in nursing. Preparation for technical nursing practice requires an associate degree or a diploma in nursing."

Diploma Programs

Diploma nursing programs are the oldest type of educational preparation developed to qualify registered nurses. Historically, they were developed within hospitals to produce nurses who would work in the hospital as students and remain there to work after graduation. Since the nursing programs provided a ready source of nursing staff for the sponsoring hospital, much of the cost was subsidized by the hospital through its charges for patient care. Student tuition and the cost of room and board were usually low in comparison to collegiate nursing programs. More recently, student tuitions have increased in many states as hospitals have become unable to subsidize the programs through the cost of patient care.

Diploma programs in nursing range from 18 to 36 months in length. They concentrate on the components of professional education with courses in nursing and the application of nursing knowledge to patient care. The programs do not require or provide a broad-based general education. Some diploma programs have their students take college-level courses in some of the sciences—chemistry, biology, microbiology, sociology and psychology. These courses may be acceptable to colleges should the graduate wish to pursue further education in nursing. While some diploma programs provide limited nursing experience in community settings, the majority of experience and education is concentrated within the hospital setting. Upon completion of the program the graduate receives a diploma from the institution and is eligible to take the state board examination for registered nurses.

After passing the examination, diploma nurses may work in any position requiring an RN license. To advance their careers, these nurses may need additional education which they can pursue through certificate programs in many specialty fields or by returning to school to earn a bachelor's degree in nursing. Recent statistics indicate that 10 percent of nurses graduating from diploma programs obtain post-RN degrees.

Educational Preparation and Advancement in Nursing

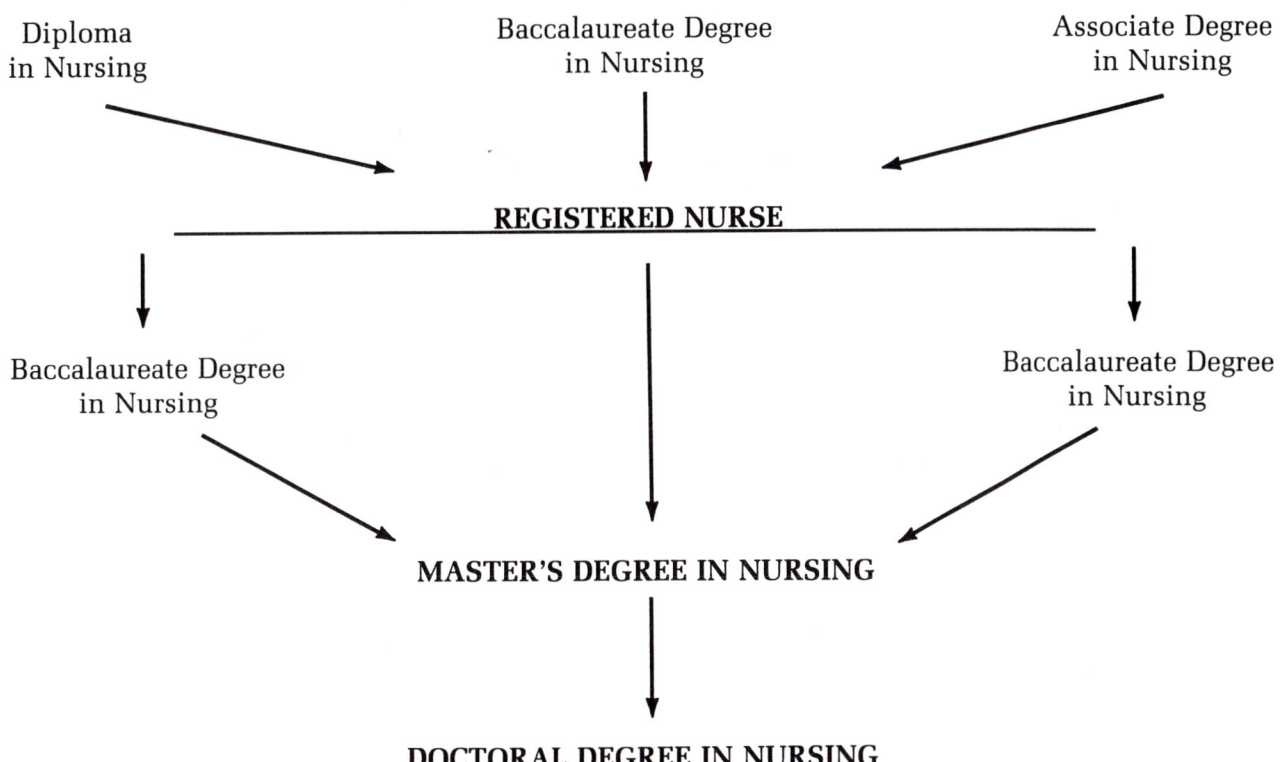

Figure 1

Associate Degree Programs

Associate degree programs in nursing were begun in the 1950s. They were developed to produce technical nurses in two years to help meet the nursing shortage. Since that time, associate degree nursing programs have proliferated more than any other type of basic nursing program. They have paralleled the growth of community colleges in the United States, and in many community colleges the associate degree nursing program enrolls the highest or second highest number of students. In addition to community colleges, associate degree nursing programs are found in four-year colleges that award associate degrees. Costs vary from the relatively inexpensive tuition of most community colleges to the higher tuitions charged by many private four-year colleges.

Associate degree nursing programs are for two full academic years. They offer some general courses as well as courses in nursing. The nursing component may include experiences in the community setting; however, the majority of nursing clinical experiences are in hospital and nursing home settings. Upon completion of the program the graduate receives an associate degree in nursing and is eligible to take the state board examination for registered nurses.

After passing the examination these nurses may work in any nursing position requiring an RN license. Should they wish to advance their careers, they too may pursue additional education through certificate programs in many of the specialty fields or a bachelor's degree in nursing. Since associate degree nursing programs have a collegiate base, many but probably not all of the courses may be applied to those needed to earn the baccalaureate degree. Recent statistics indicate that approximately seven percent of associate degree nursing graduates obtain post-RN degrees.

Baccalaureate Degree Programs

The first bachelor's degree programs in nursing were developed in the early 1900s. Nursing leaders of that time recognized that nurses needed a broad-based education in order to effectively care for people from many cultures and from diverse socioeconomic situations, races and religions. They also saw the need to have nurses become articulate advocates of their patients on matters of health care legislation and health care funding, and in developing patterns of health care delivery. Today, bachelor's degree nursing programs are found in a wide variety of public and private four-year colleges. Tuition varies from the lower costs charged by public colleges to higher tuitions charged by many private schools.

Baccalaureate degree nursing programs generally last four academic years although many students attend summer sessions and complete the program in three years. The educational focus of these programs is broad-based, containing general educational courses required by all students receiving a bachelor's degree—courses in English, the humanities, and the natural, behavioral and social sciences, as well as courses in the professional major, nursing. The courses in nursing include clinical experiences in a wide variety of settings—the hospital, nursing homes

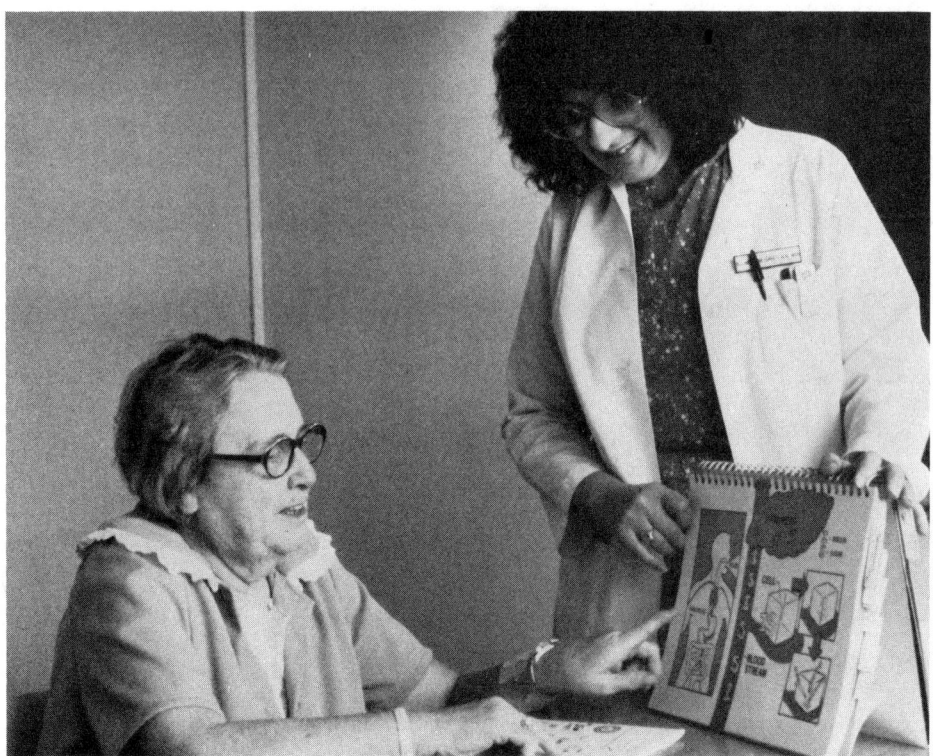
Teaching a woman about her health.

and community settings of all kinds. The amount of clinical time spent in any one setting may vary from program to program depending upon curricular orientation and the clinical facilities available in the geographical area. Many of these programs also have elective nursing courses in which students concentrate on an area of nursing they wish to work in upon graduation. Such electives may include experiences in the hospital or community, or in a specific specialty area of nursing, such as pediatrics or psychiatry.

Upon completion of the program, the graduate receives a bachelor's degree in nursing and is eligible to take the state board examination for registered nurses. After passing the examination, the nurses may work in any position requiring an RN license and those that also require a bachelor's degree. To advance their careers, they may need additional education, which they can pursue through certificate programs in many specialty fields or by returning to school to earn a master's degree in nursing. Currently, approximately 12 percent of the graduates of baccalaureate degree nursing programs obtain higher degrees.

If you are a person with a baccalaureate or higher degree in another field and are thinking about changing your career goals to nursing, this is quite possible. You will receive credit for many of the general edu-

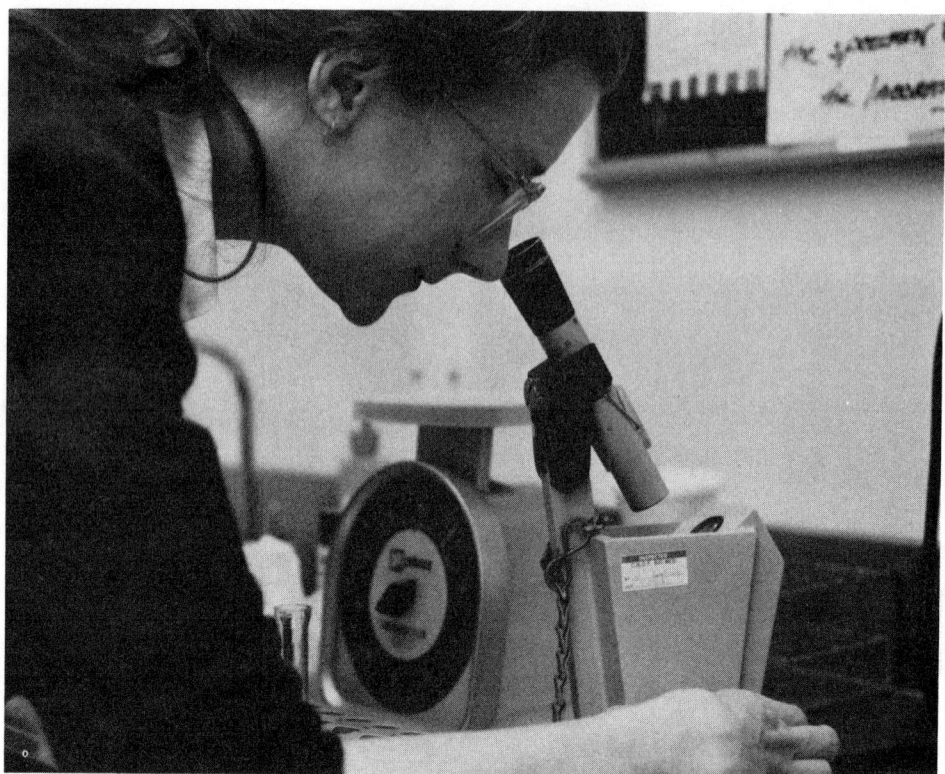
Applying knowledge in the basic sciences in clinical situations.

cation courses you have already taken. It will probably take about two years to obtain your B.S. in nursing. If you also plan to take a master's degree, you may be able to weave some of the necessary courses into the final semesters of your undergraduate study.

Master's Degree Programs

There are presently master's degree programs in nursing across the country. They build on the generalist preparation of undergraduate education in nursing. The vast majority of master's programs are found on a clinical specialty area although some feature administration or educational majors or minors. Master's degree programs vary in length from two to four semesters, depending on the area of concentration and the curriculum.

Graduate progams are for nurses who want to increase their career opportunities and assume more responsibility. A master's degree can

Introduction to Nursing and Nursing Education 9

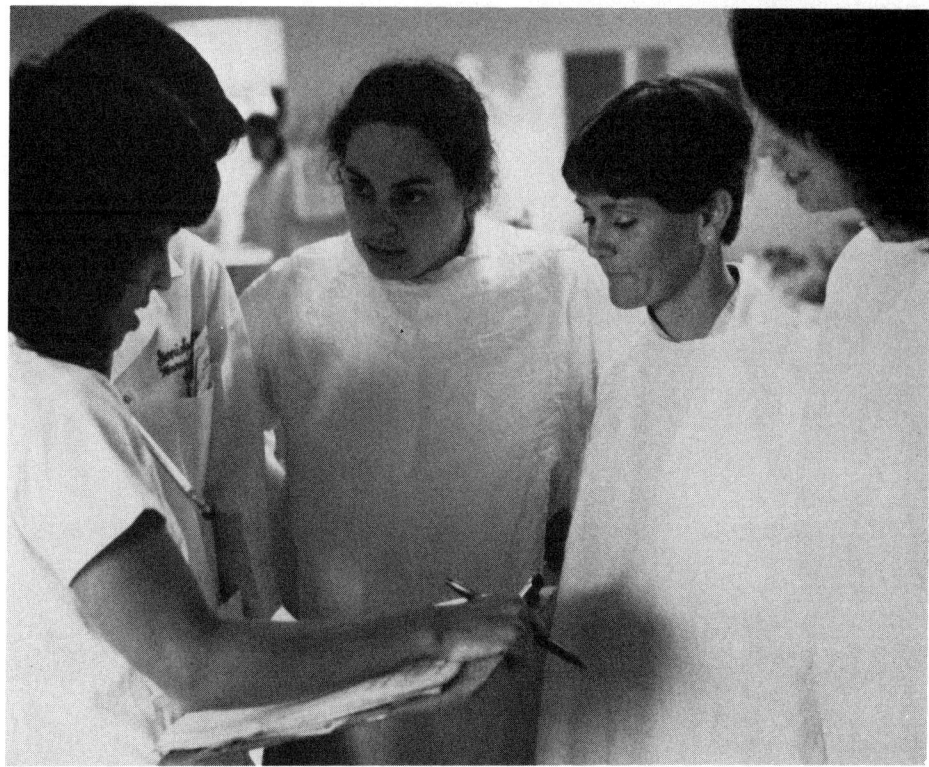

Master's degree students consulting in the clinical unit.

open up a whole new spectrum of options in teaching, research and practice. The list of specialty areas in which education can be obtained is long. Some of the possibilities are listed below but there are still many others.

CLINICAL SPECIALTIES

- Geriatrics
- Medical-surgical nursing (sub-specialties include intensive care, neurology and chronic and acute diseases)
- Midwifery
- Obstetrics and gynecology (sub-specialties include high risk perinatal care, genetic counseling and neonatology)
- Pediatrics (sub-specialties include perinatal care, mental retardation, the handicapped, intensive care, chronic and acute care and health of well children)

10   New Careers in Nursing

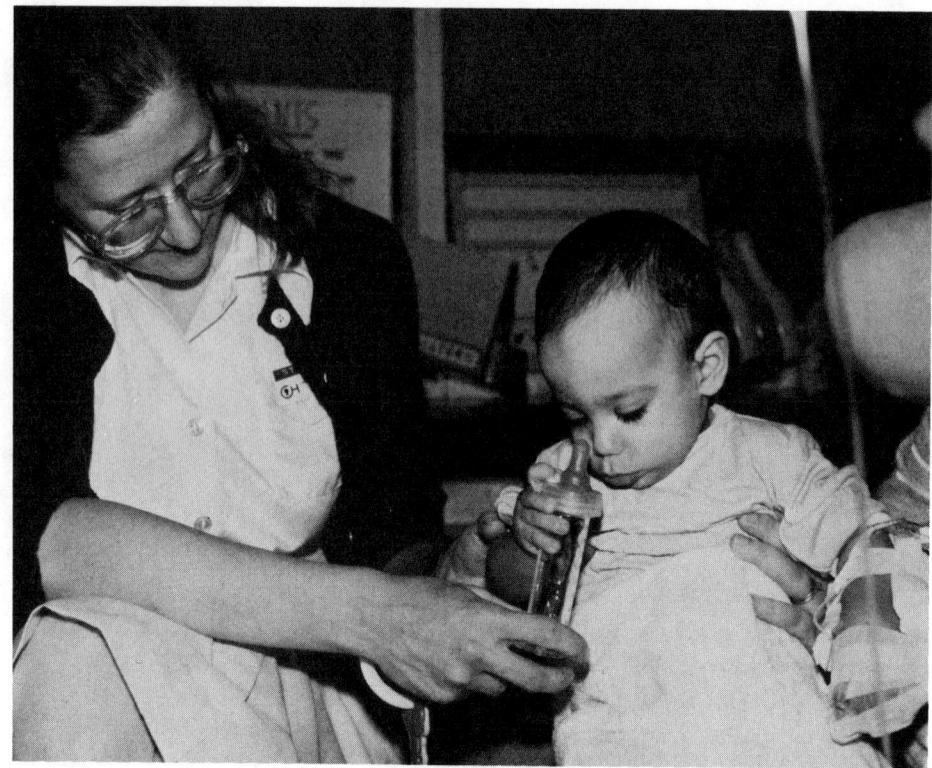

An elective course in pediatrics.

- Psychiatric-mental health (sub-specialties include the chronically mentally ill, community mental health crisis management and child psychiatry)
- Community health nursing
- School nursing
- Primary care of individuals and families

Doctoral Nursing Programs

There are currently 24 doctoral programs in nursing that accept applicants with educational preparation at the master's level. The doctoral programs are intended to develop top level leaders, researchers and scholars in the profession. The titles of the degrees vary from school to school and may be Doctor of Nursing Science(D.N.Sc.), Doctor of Education (Ed.D.) or Doctor of Philosophy (Ph.D.). The title of the degree is not as important as the quality of the school that offers it or its reputation for turning out top scholars. For some, the thought of obtaining a doctoral degree may seem farfetched. Nonetheless, since none of us know where life may lead us, it is especially important for those who have a notion of being influential in nursing to heed the guidelines that follow for choosing their educational track.

Choosing a Nursing Program

When choosing an educational program in nursing, either at the undergraduate or graduate level, choose one that meets your interests or needs—one that provides you with the credentials or degree you want, and one that will help you develop a network of nursing contacts that will aid you in your future career and job opportunities. Since you will invest a considerable amount of time, money and energy in any educational program, investigate your options carefully. When examining nursing programs, consider the following points carefully:

• *Is the program accredited by the National League for Nursing (NLN)?* The NLN is the official professional accrediting body for programs in nursing. Other educational bodies may accredit the program but cannot attest to the quality of the nursing component. Graduation from a non-NLN-accredited program may cause difficulty if you wish to pursue higher nursing education since many baccalaureate or graduate nursing programs will only accept applicants from NLN-accredited programs. Other higher degree programs may accept applicants from non-NLN-accredited programs only after evaluating each individual applicant very carefully.

• *Will graduation from the program grant you a degree in nursing?* Many educational programs are currently being marketed for RNs to complete a bachelor's degree very quickly. Many of these programs grant bachelor's degrees in fields other than nursing. Graduating from one of these will pose difficulties if you seek admission to a graduate program in nursing where a bachelor's degree in nursing is a prerequisite for admission. A few graduate nursing programs will admit students with a bachelor's degree in other fields. However, these students must complete the equivalent of most undergraduate nursing courses. In effect, students complete bachelor's work in nursing before they progress to graduate work. Graduating from a program initially that grants a bachelor's in nursing saves time, effort and money.

- *Does the program have an excellent image and reputation?* You might ask nurses you know about the program. You also might call the National League for Nursing or the American Nurses Association (or their local, state or regional organizations).

- *What is the size and quality of the program's student body?* The size of the student group should provide you with a sense of whether the program is an "educational mill" or not. The admission criteria should indicate the intellectual level of the students you will be interacting with. You might also value heterogeneity in student groups and this is another point you could explore.

- *What resources are available at the school, college or university?* You should evaluate the quality of the libraries, classrooms, study and recreational areas.

- *Does the program have excellent faculty?* Consider the academic credentials of the faculty in the program's brochure or catalogue. Determine the faculty's level of publication by reviewing the author's index in the Cumulative Index to Nursing and Allied Health Literature, which can be found in nursing and medical school libraries. You should also be interested in the level of faculty research, particularly if you are contemplating graduate education. Is faculty research consistent with your research interests? Is the faculty's research funded, and if so, by whom? You may need to talk with individual faculty members to gain this latter information. You might also want to know if the faculty are active in professional organizations and in furthering the development of the profession. Some of this information may be gleaned by reviewing the programs of the local, regional and national meetings of the American Nurses Association and other professional nursing specialty groups. Also, check whether faculty have received awards from within or outside of the profession for their involvement or leadership in behalf of the profession.

- *Do the program's best credentialed and published faculty actually teach students or are students taught by less credentialed faculty and by teaching assistants?*

- *Is there a good job market for graduates of the program you are interested in?*

- *Is the program flexible enough to meet your needs and interests?*

- *What is the cost of the program?* In addition to examining the actual direct costs, evaluate the costs of alternate programs in relation to your long-range career goals and interests. The least expensive program may end up costing you the most in time, effort and money.

- *Will the program introduce you to leaders in nursing and provide you with valuable contacts for career development and future job opportunities?*

While these are some points to consider when choosing an educational program in nursing, there are undoubtedly others that are important to you. Consider them all very carefully and spend your resources wisely.

Financing Your Education

Financing your education can be done with the help of scholarships, loans and work study. You begin inquiring about these methods of financing through your high school counselor or through the financial aid office of the school to which you are applying. Financial aid is usually awarded based on need. Other children in the family, a mother or father who is also a student, the distance the student must travel to school, total family income and debt are factors that are considered in the awarding of aid.

Scholarship aid is available from private, state and federal funds. Colleges and universities often have scholarships financed through their endowments or established by wealthy alumni. Many civic and service organizations, such as the American Legion, Rotary, Kwanis clubs or business and church groups, sponsor scholarships. The Army and Air Force sponsor scholarships for those interested in nursing. The Army offers a four-year scholarship to eligible high school students interested in studying nursing in a baccalaureate degree program. Scholarship benefits begin in the fall semester of the student's freshman year and include full tuition, fees, books and a $100 stipend per month for expenses. Upon graduation the nurse is commissioned as a second lieutenant and is obligated to serve four years of active duty in the U.S. Army Nurse Corps. To be eligible for the scholarship, students must apply no later than December 1 of their senior year in high school. The Air Force offers a similar two-year scholarship with students applying in their sophomore year in college. Upon graduation the nurse is commissioned and is obligated for two years of active duty as an Air Force officer.

Increasingly, in an effort to fill their nursing positions, hospitals are offering scholarships to high school or college students interested in pursuing nursing as a career. Often a sum of money is awarded to a school of nursing to be applied toward the student's tuition. The scholarship grant may be for two to four years and, upon graduation, the nurse is obligated to work at the hospital for a period of consecutive months and often is assigned to a hospital unit most in need of nurses. For many years hospitals have provided tuition reimbursement plans for registered nurses who were working toward bachelor's or master's degrees. Only in the recent past have grants been awarded to those individuals pursuing basic education to become a registered nurse.

In addition to private scholarships and grants, many states offer a variety of scholarships and the federal government has offered Pell and Supplementary Educational Opportunity Grants.

Low interest loans are also available to finance your education. A maximum of $2,500 is available through guaranteed student loans available from your local bank. Federal nursing student loans are also possibilities. Some hospitals have established programs in which they will pay off a nurse's guaranteed student loan if the nurse works at the institution for a specified period of time while earning full salary.

A third option in financing your education is a work-study program. Here college students work in a variety of jobs at the college for approximately 10 hours per week and receive money that can be used for books and for living expenses. To learn more about the options that might be available to you, talk with your high school guidance counselor or college financial aid officer, or contact the National League for Nursing, or your American Nurses Association state office (see appendix I).

How to Get Started

If you are interested in pursuing nursing as a possible career, there are several ways you can investigate the field in depth. You can discuss nursing with your guidance counselor, volunteer at a local hospital for work as a candy striper, contact the National League for Nursing (or its local unit in your area) or your state's American Nurses Association office (see Appendix I, page 159).

Most high school guidance counselors are familiar with nursing as a career choice and usually have nursing contacts with whom you can talk in the local region and state. Your counselor may also arrange trips to local nursing schools for small groups interested in pursuing the discipline. Nursing representatives may also be invited to your high school to tell you more about nursing and its various programs and career options. Because nursing has changed so rapidly in the past decade, many high school counselors are unaware of the current differences in basic entry nursing programs, in advanced educational opportunities and in the many career options currently available. They may also be unaware of the career possibilities nursing currently offers for men.

Additional information on the various nursing programs, their purposes and objectives is available through the National League for Nursing in New York. By writing or telephoning the League you can obtain brochures and information on various nursing programs in your local and regional area, as well as nationally. You may also be referred to the local or state chapter of the League where you can talk with local representatives about nursing in your area.

You can also gain much information about nursing and its many career options by contacting the American Nurses Association (ANA) in Kansas City, MO, or by talking with leaders in your local or state nurse's association. Unlike the National League for Nursing, whose membership is composed of nurses and non-nurses, the American Nurses Association is only composed of nurses. Increasingly, local and state nurses associations of the ANA are receiving requests from high school students and others interested in pursuing nursing. In response to these requests, many of the chapters have developed a list of nurse volunteers who are willing to talk to groups or individuals interested in nursing or to have them visit places where nurses are employed.

Another way those interested in nursing have investigated the field is by volunteering as a candy striper in a local hospital. As a volunteer, you can gain experience working with patients and familiarize yourself with the hospital environment and its pace. You can also have contact with many members of the health care team and the opportunity to talk with nurses working in a variety of jobs who have different educational backgrounds. While this can be an excellent opportunity to explore nursing in a hospital, remember that approximately 40 percent of nurses work in settings other than hospitals. You might, on your own or through contacting a local or state nurses' association, volunteer your services in another setting and explore what nurses do elsewhere.

Do talk to nurses who live in your community about what they do and about how satisfied they are. In particular, read some of the nursing literature and find out whether any of the authors live in your area. Don't be bashful; they will, as a rule, be happy to talk to you about your future plans.

For Further Information

Write:

American Nurses Association
2420 Pershing Road
Kansas City, MO 64108

National League for Nursing
10 Columbus Circle
New York, NY 10019

Read:

Allen, V. and Sutton, C. "Associate Degree Nursing Education: Past, Present and Future." *Nursing and Health Care* 2: 496, 1981.

Associate Degree Education for Nursing 1979–1980.
    National League for Nursing
    Publication No. 23-1309

Baccalaureate Education in Nursing: Key to a Professional Career in Nursing.
    National League for Nursing
    Publication No. 15-1311

Brower, H. "Potential Advantages and Hazards of Non-traditional Education for Nurses." *Nursing and Health Care* 3:268, 1982.

A Case for Baccalaureate Preparation in Nursing.
    American Nurses Association
    Publication No. NE 6

Doctoral Programs in Nursing 1979–1980.
    National League for Nursing
    Publication No. 15-1448

Education for Nursing: The Diploma Way—1979–80.
  National League for Nursing
  Publication No. 16-1314

Enrolling in a Baccalaureate Program in Nursing.
  American Nurses Association
  Kansas City, MO, 1980

Facts About Nursing 80–81.
  American Nurses Association
  American Journal of Nursing Company
  New York, NY, 1981

Fagin, C. "Nursing as an Alternative to High Cost Care." *American Journal of Nursing* 82:56, 1982.

Funding Nursing Education.
  American Nurses Association
  Publication No. NE 7

Huckstadt, A. "Work/Study: A Bridge to Practice." *American Journal of Nursing* 81: 726, 1981.

Master's Education in Nursing: Route to Opportunities in Contemporary Nursing 1979–80.
  National League for Nursing
  Publication No. 15-1312

New Directions for Nursing in the 80's.
  American Nurses Association
  Publication No. G-147

Nursing Data Book 1981.
  National League for Nursing
  Publication No. 19-1882
  New York, NY, 1981

Nursing 81 Career Directory.
  Intermed Communications
  Horsham, PA, 1981

Palmer, I. "Florence Nightingale and International Origins of Modern Nursing." *Image* 13:28, 1981.

Perry, S. "A Doctorate—Necessary but Not Sufficient." *Nursing Outlook* 30: 95, 1982.

Practical Nursing Career—1980.
    National League for Nursing
    Publication No. 38-1328

Scholarships and Loans for Beginning Education in Nursing.
    National League for Nursing
    Publication No. 41-410

Scholarships, Fellowships, Educational Grants and Loans for Registered Nurses.
    National League for Nursing
    Publication No. 41-408

Smith, F. "Florence Nightingale: Early Feminist." *American Journal of Nursing* 81:1020, 1981.

State-Approved Schools of Nursing RN 1981.
    National League for Nursing
    New York, NY, 1981

2.

Hospitals

Modern hospitals currently employ about two-thirds of all nurses in practice. Working in a hospital can be exciting, challenging and sometimes frustrating. It is the setting that has been most highly popularized in the media and the one with which most people associate nursing. Unfortunately, the media sometimes convey a false picture of the nurse as someone who does what the physician says must be done and who is overworked and underpaid. Rarely do they stress the incredible variety of patients to whom you can give care or the wealth of job opportunities that are available.

In addition to giving direct care to patients as a staff nurse, you can choose to manage nursing care in a nursing administrative position. Inservice education programs offer you the chance to teach patients and new graduate nurses. As a clinical specialist, you can combine teaching and direct care with consultation to other nurses, physicians and various members of the health team. Research positions are also available that allow you to study nursing problems and ways to improve patient care.

But this is only the beginning. In addition to having a range of positions to choose from, you also can determine the type of patient you are most interested in caring for. You can work directly with families who are about to have a baby in a labor and delivery unit, with children and adolescents on a pediatric unit, or with adults on a medical or surgical unit. In addition you could work in a psychiatric unit, where people of all ages with emotional problems are admitted. There are also a variety of specialty areas such as the operating room, and medical, surgical, cardiac or newborn intensive care units, and kidney dialysis sites. Some of the other possibilities are the emergency room, a short-term care unit, and specialty or ambulatory care settings.

Staff Nursing

As a staff nurse you will provide direct care to patients. The age of the patients and the types of illnesses or health needs they have will vary depending on where you work. A standard work week is 40 hours, eight hours a day. You may work the day, evening or night shift permanently or rotate shifts every few weeks. Many hospitals are currently trying out flexible schedules that include four 10-hour shifts followed by three days off, or three 12-hour shifts per week. You can expect to work weekends, but the number per month will vary, depending upon the number of nurses on the unit, the hospital policy and the unit's needs and scheduling patterns. A typical day for a staff nurse will vary greatly depending upon the illness levels and ages of the patients.

To qualify as a staff nurse, you must be licensed as an LPN or R.N. in the state where you practice. Of course, this means that you first must obtain the required educational preparation to sit for the examination. Staff nurses in a hospital may advance their careers in a number of ways. Some hospitals have levels of staff positions. Staff nurses remain at the bedside giving direct patient care, and as their clinical care skills, education and contributions to improving direct care increase, they advance to higher staff nurse levels. With each successive level, salaries increase as well.

Some staff nurses decide their interest is in teaching and many seek positions in in-service education. Others advance their careers by following an administrative route as head nurse, supervisor, assistant director, director of nursing or vice president for hospital administration (see Figure 2, page 59). Career advancement for nurses in a hospital is exceedingly wide open for ambitious, energetic, career-minded individuals. It should be remembered, however, that advanced education will probably be required to move up the career ladder.

Salaries vary a great deal for nurses working within a hospital. Depending upon the geographical location of the hospital, staff nurse salaries range from $16,000 to $24,000. Salaries for directors of nursing range from $25,000 to $65,000.

On a Surgical Unit

Work on a surgical unit is usually fast paced. It requires quick thinking and decision-making and the ability to withstand stress and organize work so that people can be helped to undergo needed treatment despite their fear, discomfort and, often, pain.

A day for a staff nurse on an adult surgical unit may include preparing patients for upcoming surgery. This may begin several days ahead of time and involve helping the patient through a series of tests and other diagnostic procedures. As the time for the actual operation approaches, the nurse will make sure the patient understands the nature of the surgery, what can be anticipated during the course of recovery and how to reduce discomfort. For instance, this might mean teaching a patient the correct way to deep breathe and cough, and to splint chest or abdominal muscles to minimize pain. It may be necessary to explain equipment that will be used, procedures to be done and drugs to be taken during the postoperative period. To accomplish these tasks well, the nurse must be completely familiar with equipment and operative routines, and also sensitive to the patient's physiological and emotional states. Many patients in the preoperative period are weak from their conditions and feel threatened by the thought of what needs to be done as a remedy. Thus, teaching needs to be carefully paced, and carried out in a supportive manner. On the day of surgery, the nurse will make sure all is ready, including the consent forms and results of the patient's blood work and laboratory studies. The patient must be checked for proper clothing and for temperature, pulse, respiration and blood pressure to be sure they are within a normal range. Following this, preoperative medications will be administered and the patient sent to surgery.

On return from surgery, the nurse must be alert for changes in blood pressure, pulse and respiration. The surgical site must be carefully observed for signs of bleeding. The patient will need help to change positions and breathe deeply to prevent pneumonia from developing. These position changes will also help improve circulation and prevent formation of blood clots. During this time the patient may require transfusions, infusions and medications for pain relief. As you can imagine, it is a time when everyone must be on their toes.

On any given day, a nurse in a surgical unit will care for one or more patients who are recovering from surgery performed several days ago. These patients may need to be assisted in bathing or dressing, getting out of bed and in moving about and walking increasing amounts each day. The nurse will typically change dressings, cleanse and observe wounds, administer medications and intravenous solutions and spend time charting or recording what was done for each patient. Plans of care for each patient will need to be updated and plans developed for discharge. The latter may involve teaching or consultation with the patient's family regarding care and activity at home. During a typical day, the nurse will also consult with physicians, dieticians and, possibly, social service personnel about the care of patients.

Nurses in surgical units have identified some of the most satisfying aspects of their work as seeing patients arrive in pain with acute emergencies, receive treatment or surgery and be discharged feeling well within a week or two. The technical skills involved in caring for many patients appeal to nurses who enjoy working with equipment and machines as well as with people. Nurses mention the most frustrating aspect of their work to be the limited time they have to spend with each patient because the units tend to be very busy. Often patients are discharged within a week, depending upon the type of surgery, which limits contact even more. The other frustrating aspect often cited is the amount of recording and other paperwork.

CHARACTERISTICS IMPORTANT FOR THIS TYPE OF WORK INCLUDE:

- ability to handle stress
- skill in helping others cope with stress
- quick thinking and decision-making
- ability to organize work

Operating Room

In addition to assisting physicians with surgery, OR nurses often visit patients prior to surgery and help them understand the reason for the surgery and what they may anticipate their postoperative period will be like. They also do preoperative and postoperative teaching.

Neurosurgery

One operating room nurse explained her interest in this area of nursing as the excitement and pace of the operating room, the interest and confidence of the people working there and her interest in the technical side of nursing. Also, by working in a large OR department she was able to remain in the specialty area she enjoys most—neurosurgery. The following is a description of her day.*

---

*"Interview: Laurie Dean." *Today's OR Nurse* 3:30, 1982.

Hospitals 23

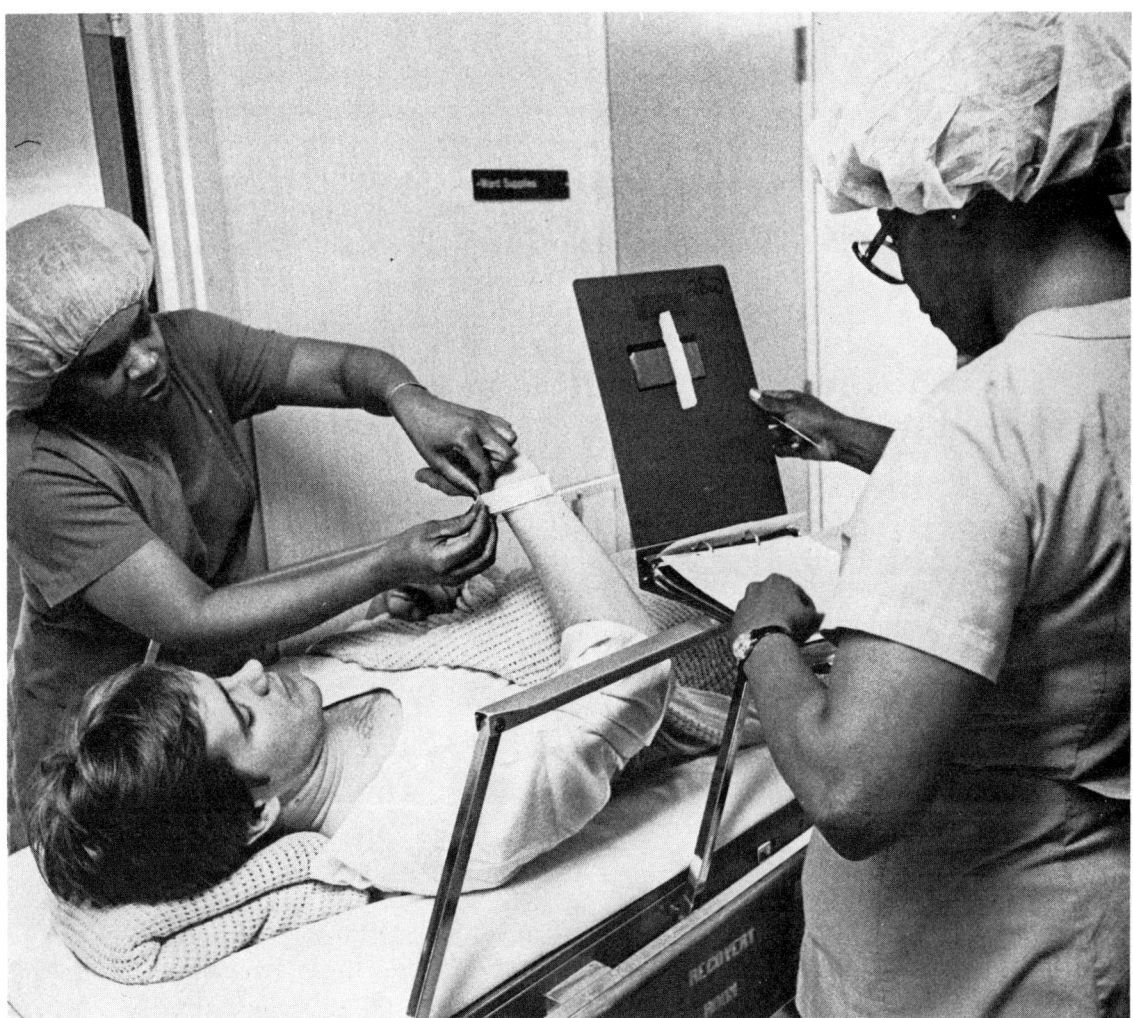

Nurses checking identification tag and reviewing medical chart before surgery. (Photo courtesy of the Veterans Administration)

After reporting to the OR at 7:45 A.M., she is assigned either to scrub or to circulate on a neurosurgical operation at 8 A.M. Many times she will have visited the patient the previous day. If she is assigned as a scrub nurse, she will scrub her hands for surgery and don a sterile gown. She will then help the physicians put on their sterile gloves, and assist in draping the patient for surgery. During the surgical procedure, she passes sterile instruments to the physician, holds retractors to keep the operative area clearly visible or assists in other ways. If she is to circulate during the operation, her task is to help position the patient for surgery and to make sure the consent form, labo-

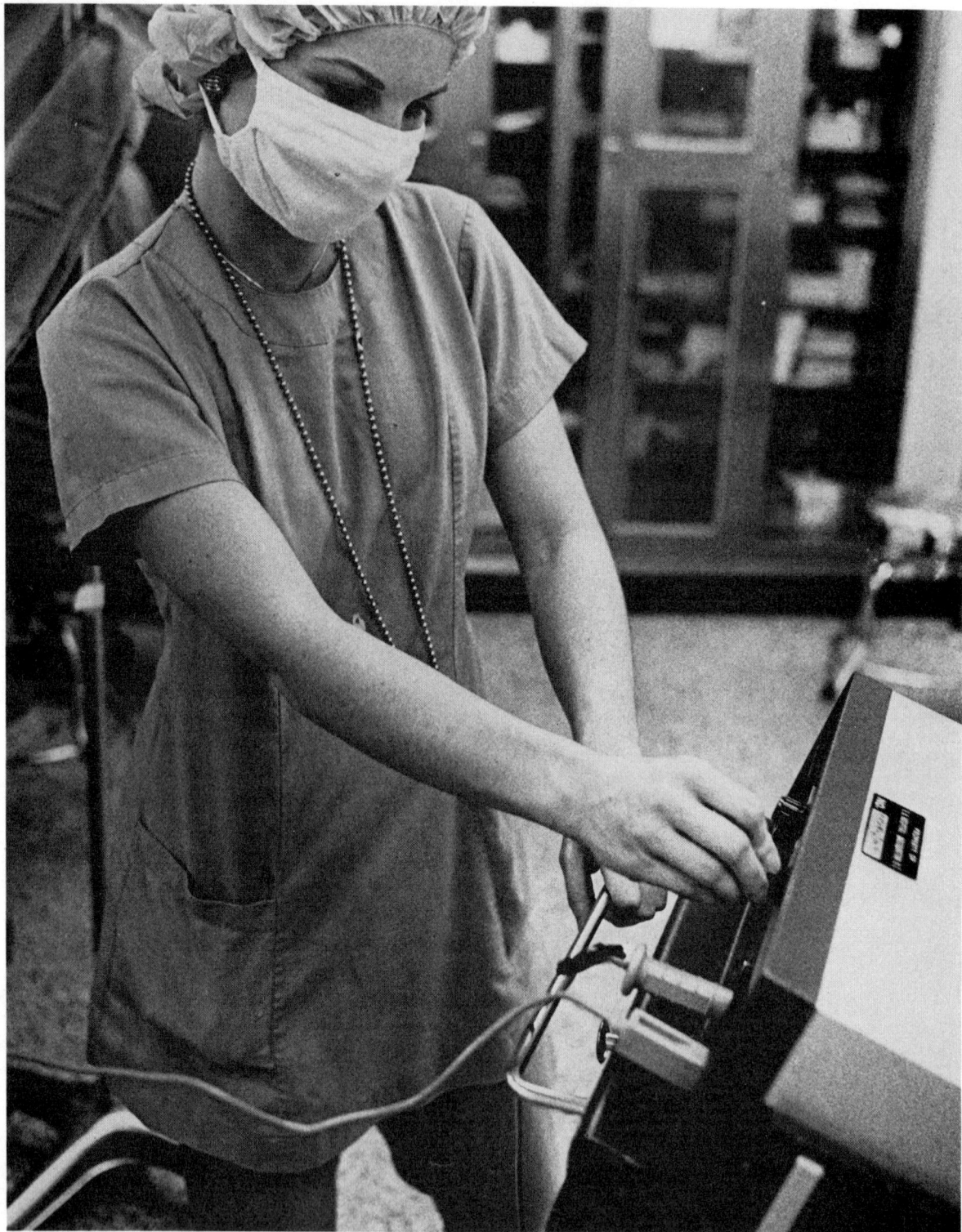
Testing equipment to be used on a patient in surgery. (Photo courtesy of the Veterans Administration)

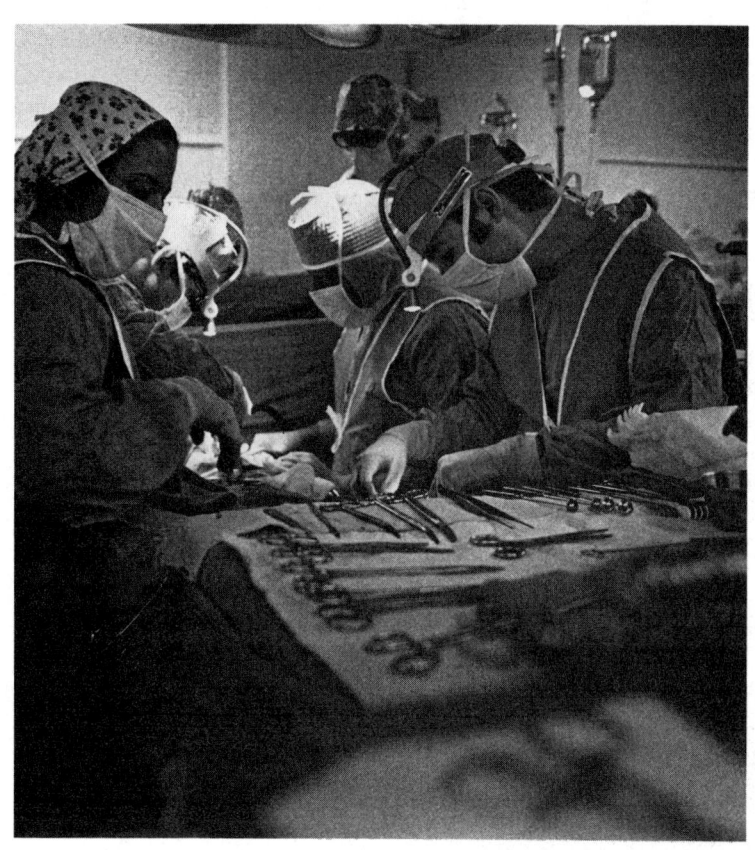

Working in the operating room.

ratory studies and other necessary paperwork are complete. Once surgery begins, she drops sterile sponges, additional instruments and supplies on the scrub nurse's table. Later, she helps with the sponge counts to make sure all the ones used have been accounted for. Since many operations are long and tedious, the nurse usually scrubs once or twice a day for periods up to six hours. On rare occasions, it may be longer. If she circulates, she may attend several operations in one day.

Later in the afternoon, after she has finished scrubbing or circulating, she visits patients facing surgery the following day. She also visits as many patients postoperatively as she can, especially those whose surgery was particularly long or difficult.

The nurse emphasized the importance of team effort between physicians and nurses, especially during the surgery. While there is much tension, the tension is focused on the patient and the procedure that is being done. She explained that many neurosurgical operations begin with regular-sized instruments, until the surgeon opens the patient's skull or bony spinal column. From this point on, the surgery is performed under a microscope used by the surgeon. The room lights are turned off so that the intensity of the microscope light is better. As the surgeon operates, the scrub nurse watches a TV video system that is hooked up to the microscope so that she can see what the surgeon is doing and can anticipate what instruments will be needed next.

The nurse also commented on the incredible amount of technology that has been developed over the years for use in neurosurgery. One example is an ultrasound device used to vibrate and shatter tumors into minuscule pieces that can then be removed by suctioning. The device can be regulated for use on substances such as bone. Part of her excitement with neurosurgical OR nursing is the use of advanced technology that helps improve a patient's recovery and outcome.

Day Surgery Unit

Ambulatory or day surgery is a service provided to patients so they do not remain overnight in the hospital as inpatients. The service is growing rapidly as efforts are made to control the costs of health care and as physicians and consumers become more knowledgeable about and comfortable with this type of arrangement. In a recent survey conducted by the American Hospital Association, 70 percent of the hospitals surveyed nationwide now offer ambulatory services. The day surgery being performed includes procedures such as tonsillectomies, extraction of teeth, breast biopsies and surgical repair of old scars.

One group of staff nurses working in a day surgery unit share their roles in the following way. Each month is broken into two-week periods. For one two-week period a portion of the nurses work in the recovery room caring for patients immediately after surgery. For the other two weeks they function as primary nurses. Their responsibilities in this role encompass admitting their patients, circulating for their operations and discharging the patients later in the day. When admitting patients they perform a physical and psychological assessment and begin educating patients about their condition: what to expect during surgery and the followup care needed after discharge. The primary nurse assesses, evaluates and supports the patient during the surgery. Following surgery, the primary nurse continues to monitor the patient, working with the recovery room nurse. The primary nurse is responsible for ensuring that the patient and family understand all postoperative instructions. In addition, primary nurses make a telephone followup call to their patients the day following surgery to evaluate their postoperative status, reactions and adjustments at home. This group of nurses chose to rotate between their roles as primary nurses and recovery room nurses every two weeks because they find the role of primary nurse in this setting to be exhausting. By rearranging their roles into two-week segments, they feel they are provided with a fulfilling and challenging role as well as one that will avoid burnout.*

Nurses working in operating room units have identified some of the most satisfying aspects of the work as including seeing patients improve rapidly following their surgery, and the feeling of camaraderie between members of the operating room team. Frustrating aspects of the work include surgery that is not successful, finding unexpected terminal illnesses in patients during surgery and sometimes much paperwork when circulating.

CHARACTERISTICS IMPORTANT FOR THIS TYPE OF WORK INCLUDE:

- ability to handle stress
- satisfaction in performing technical skills
- satisfaction in needing to see patients only for short periods of time

Emergency Room

Nurses in these units need to be prepared for a variety of patient problems and to be able to make decisions and act upon them immediately. Patients arriving in an emergency room can be in grave condition due to accidents, cardiac arrest, assault or rape. In some cases they may be unconscious. Then there are abandoned children, people with broken limbs and animal bites, and patients who have taken drug overdoses. The variety of problems is endless.

"There is no 'typical' day when you work as a staff nurse in an emergency room (ER)," commented one staff nurse in such a unit. Some days are quiet except for a few minor trauma cases, a broken bone, a person suffering from a heart attack, a few people with colds or the flu who

---

*Camp, M. A. "Change to Primary Care in Day Surgery." AORN Journal 34:342, 1981.

have no family doctor and who use the emergency room to make up for it. Then there are other days when a major disaster may have taken place in a local industrial plant or when there has been a bus accident or other catastrophe in the region. Think about being an ER nurse when Mount St. Helens erupted. That's when the ER really becomes hectic.

The ER nurse is the first health team person the patient usually encounters in the emergency room. The nurse interviews patients, evaluates their condition and identifies their immediate needs before sending them to the ER secretary for registration. If a patient's needs are urgent, registration is delayed until after they have been treated. After the nurse evaluates the patient's condition and after registration, the patient is shown to one of the treatment areas in the emergency room to be examined and treated by a physician. This process, called triage (from a French verb meaning to sort), determines who can wait a bit and who needs immediate treatment, and is only one part of the ER staff nurse's role.

ER nurses must recognize life threatening emergencies and apply their knowledge and skills to intervene effectively. This means continually assessing and monitoring patients in the unit. Teaching health care to patients and families, prevention of accidents and followup care are also important aspects of the nurse's role, as referral of patients to community and social services is important to recovery.

This is how things usually happen in the ER, but occasionally the sequence is disrupted. Recently, a staff nurse shared an experience that occurred after three commuter trains collided during the morning rush hour fairly near a Philadelphia hospital. More than 400 people were eventually sent to area hospitals. Within 15 minutes of the accident more than a dozen patients arrived at the emergency room. For the next two hours a stream of patients, relatives, reporters, policemen and railroad officials poured through the emergency room doors. The ER clerical supervisor registered patients as they arrived. As the census grew, it became apparent that the train accident was more serious than had initially been anticipated. Additional nurses, x-ray technicians and other staff were called to transport patients from other hospital units and ER staff nurses were called in from home. By noon more than 60 patients had been treated and released—four patients had been hospitalized. The entire health care team responded quickly and efficiently. To outside observers, the ER that morning may have looked confused, but in reality everyone knew what to do and did it. That day, however, health teaching and some community referrals were overlooked!*

Nurses working in emergency rooms have identified some of the most

---

*"HUP Response to Train Disaster." *HUP Date*, p. 4, October 29, 1979.

satisfying aspects of their work as being able to decrease the pain and panic of patients who have arrived in acute pain or distress and treating them so they can leave, feeling better, in a short time. Other satisfying aspects mentioned include the fast pace, excitement and variety of problems encountered. Nurses mention the frustrating aspects to include the amount of paperwork and occasional feelings of exhaustion.

CHARACTERISTICS IMPORTANT FOR THIS TYPE OF WORK INCLUDE:

- ability to handle stress
- ability to help others cope with stress
- ability to make decisions quickly
- satisfaction in needing to see patients only for brief periods of time

Surgical Intensive Care Unit

A surgical intensive care unit looks like the busy hospital units of many television shows. These units contain a mass of scientific equipment, including video screens for monitoring heart rates, blood pressures and respirations, and what appears to an outsider to be a bewildering array of bottles, tubes and machines. Physicians, respiratory therapists, laboratory technicians and nurses are constantly attending to acutely ill patients while buzzers ring out to signal anything from a heart that has stopped beating to a patient's rise in blood pressure. This type of environment, with its challenge, fast pace and accompanying tension, is one that may appeal to you.

Nurses in surgical intensive care units usually care for only one or two patients a day because of the acuteness of their conditions. The types of patients found in these units range from those recovering from open heart surgery, and from removal of all or parts of major body organs, to those suffering from major accidents or other trauma. One nurse described a recent typical day in one such unit.

> Upon arriving on the unit the nurse was assigned to care for a man who had been admitted two hours earlier from open heart surgery. He was still unconscious from anesthesia, and she was

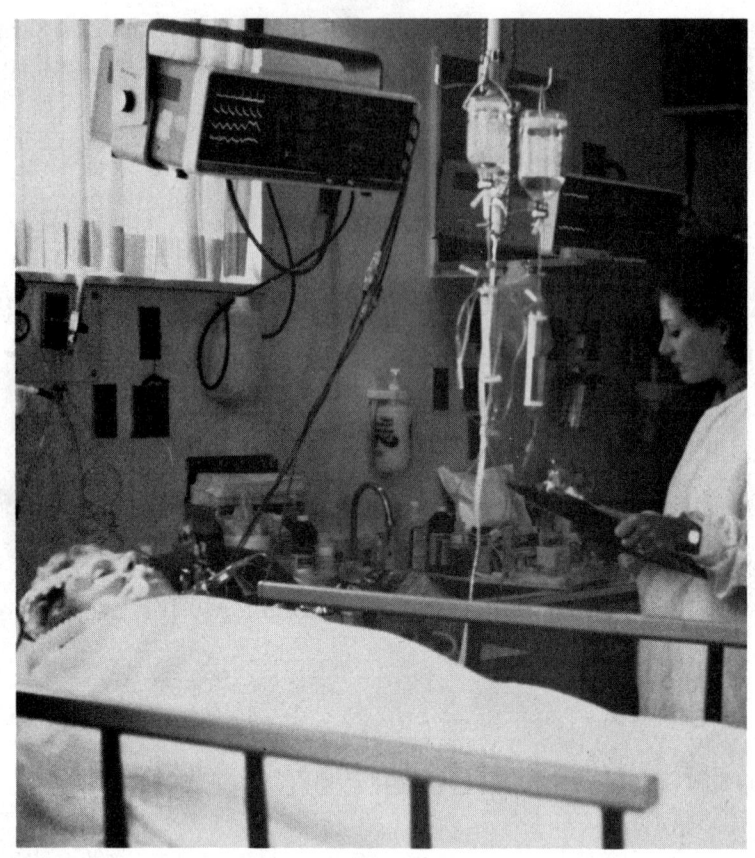

Working in surgical intensive care.

responsible for monitoring the fluids and intravenous drugs he was receiving, as well as his breathing rate, blood pressure, heart rate, urine output and body temperature. She was also responsible for being alert to signs of potential emergencies, such as irregular heart rates.

For the first two hours of the eight-hour shift the nurse carefully monitored the man's breathing, heart rate and blood pressure. When his blood pressure increased, a dangerous sign, she increased the intravenous dose of the cardiac medication. After a little over two hours, flashing lights and alarms indicated the man had regained consciousness. The nurse then told him where he was and how well he was doing. When the man indicated he had pain, she asked several questions to determine where the pain was coming from and the reason for it. Because his response indicated potential danger, she ordered an electrocardiogram be taken. The doctor in charge evaluated the tracing and ordered an increased dose of one medication which was intended to stabilize the heart rate pattern. When the man responded well to the medication, the nurse and anesthesiologist

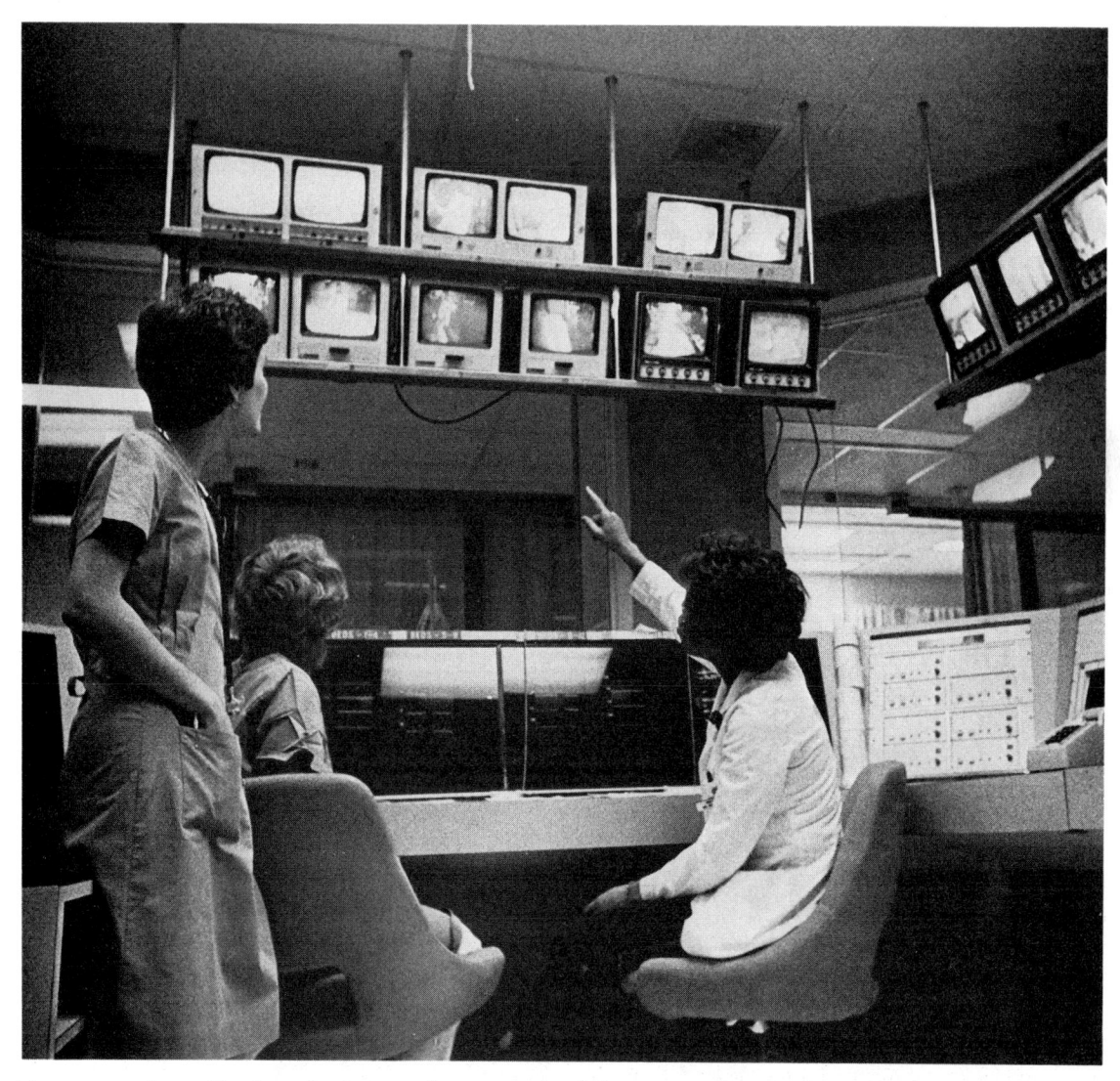

Nurses and medical technician observe television consoles and patient monitors in an intensive care unit. (Photo courtesy of the Veterans Administration)

removed the respirator which the patient had been dependent on for breathing and replaced it with an oxygen mask. The nurse then asked the man's wife, who was in the waiting room, if she would like to visit her husband. As the woman visited her husband, the nurse observed them both for signs of emotional stress. Later, she used these observations in an important part of her work—to help the wife and patient talk about their concerns and try to relax.

After the wife's short visit, the nurse and anesthesiologist taught the man breathing exercises to help keep his lungs inflated and to prevent pneumonia. For the remaining hours of the shift the nurse carefully monitored the man's vital signs, intravenous fluids, signs of postoperative complications and pain. Should an emergency have occurred, quick decision-making would have been needed.*

As a nurse working in this type of unit, you will use many technical skills and work with much equipment and many machines. Nurses mention the challenge, excitement and satisfaction of helping patients and their families through critical situations as positive aspects of this type of work. The most frustrating aspects of the work cited by nurses include short staffing, malfunctioning equipment and emergency situations that end unsuccessfully.

CHARACTERISTICS IMPORTANT FOR THIS TYPE OF WORK INCLUDE:

- ability to handle stress
- ability to make accurate decisions and act quickly
- interest in working with your hands and with equipment

Psychiatric Unit

Working in a psychiatric unit can be pleasant and restful at one time and tense, depressing and exhausting at another. Patients in these units have difficulty functioning in society outside the hospital. The psychiatric unit offers a safe, therapeutic environment in which patients can begin to learn or relearn acceptable, helpful behavior and independent functioning. A nurse's role in these units requires setting limits on be-

---

*Harris, A. "HUP Nurse Monitors Intensive Care Ward." *Daily Pennsylvanian* (Philadelphia, PA), p. 1, April 8, 1982.

havior, behavioral role modeling for patients, and helping patients learn to function independently and to cooperate with others. Caring for patients in a psychiatric unit requires fewer technical skills than work in many other units and more skills in communication, counseling individuals and families, and group process.

Patients who are admitted to psychiatric units are often confused and afraid and many have difficulty carrying out basic activities of daily living. A nurse's day might begin by helping one or more patients bathe, dress and perform their usual morning hygiene. The aim of care is to progressively guide the patients in assuming more responsibility for their own care so that they can return to society. To that end, the nurse may guide patients on a unit to organize, plan and share activities that demonstrate self-control, cooperation and the ability to complete tasks successfully.

The nurse might attend and participate in patient government meetings, where plans for special activities, such as holiday parties or trips, are planned, and where the appropriateness of each patient's behavior can be evaluated by other patients. The nurse might help patients plan their daily schedule and participate in special activities, such as baking, playing cards or other games with groups of patients; and she may accompany patients on trips outside the hospital to museums, movies, sports events and picnics. Here again, the object of the activity is to help patients focus their thoughts, participate and cooperate with each other, assume responsibility for their actions and begin to function independently once again.

During the course of the day the nurse may lead or participate in group therapy sessions by guiding patients' conversation in realistic directions or by helping keep the session on target. The nurses also dispense medications, develop patient care plans and record their observations on each patient's chart. Part of each day is spent consulting with doctors, social workers, and recreational or occupational therapists on the behavior and progress of the group of patients they care for. Since the problems of patients are often entwined with those of their families, the nurse may also meet with the patient and family together to help them develop insight into the ways they interact as a group.

Nurses say that the most satisfying aspects of work in a psychiatric unit include seeing patients improve behaviorally and become responsible and independent upon discharge. These nurses enjoy the collegial relationships they are able to develop with other members of the health team and the opportunity to use interpersonal skills in a therapeutic way. The frustrating part of their work is often their inability to affect social conditions that contribute to readmission. It can be discouraging to see patients return to the hospital again and again, despite all of their effort.

CHARACTERISTICS IMPORTANT FOR THIS TYPE OF WORK INCLUDE:

- emotional stability and maturity
- ability to tolerate unusual behavior
- insight and interest in behavior
- good communication skills
- ability to listen
- ability to tolerate delayed rewards

Labor and Delivery Unit

Working in a labor and delivery unit can be one of the most exciting yet tension producing settings in which you might ever work. The experiences of your day can leave you on an emotional high as you share with a couple the birth of a wanted, healthy infant. Even nurses who have worked in these units for years continue to share the warm, happy feeling of each couple's excitement about their newborn. Unfortunately, there are times when the birth of a defective or stillborn infant can leave you feeling very depressed. Tension can build when a fetus or mother encounters problems and emergency measures and fast action on your part can make the difference between a live or stillborn infant. However, these periods occur far less frequently than the periods of pleasant excitement.

A nurse's day in a labor and delivery unit typically involves providing care to a woman or couple during labor. The nurse provides physical care such as back rubs, sponge baths and mouth hygiene to the laboring woman. The woman's temperature, pulse, respiration, blood pressure, fetal heart rate and uterine contractions must be evaluated. Women may need to be taught breathing techniques or other methods to cope with the discomfort that arises as labor progresses. Both the woman and her husband will require reassurance and support that all is going as it should. The nurse also administers medications for pain relief, gives or monitors intravenous solutions, and evaluates fetal status and the woman's contractions through the use of fetal monitoring. Depending upon the setting, the nurse may perform vaginal examinations to determine how the woman's labor is progressing.

The nurse may remain with the couple during delivery of their infant, depending upon the length of labor. Here the nurse helps position the woman on the delivery table or in bed, readies the equipment needed for the birth and care of the infant and explains to the mother and father, if he is present, what is happening. As soon as the baby is born, the nurse provides immediate care to the newborn. This includes clearing the infant's airway of mucus, cleansing its eyes, footprinting and applying an identification bracelet. The infant must be kept warm and dry, weighed and have a clamp or tie put on the umbilical cord. The nurse may perform a brief physical examination of the infant to determine its general condition and to identify whether it is full term, premature or past term. Following delivery, the same nurse may care for the mother in the recovery room before the mother is transferred to the maternity floor. In a small hospital, the same nurse may work in the labor, delivery, nursery and postpartum unit during the same day or week, or may rotate through these units on a schedule.

The nurse working in a labor and delivery unit may also be involved with cesarean births. She may be the scrub nurse (the nurse who passes

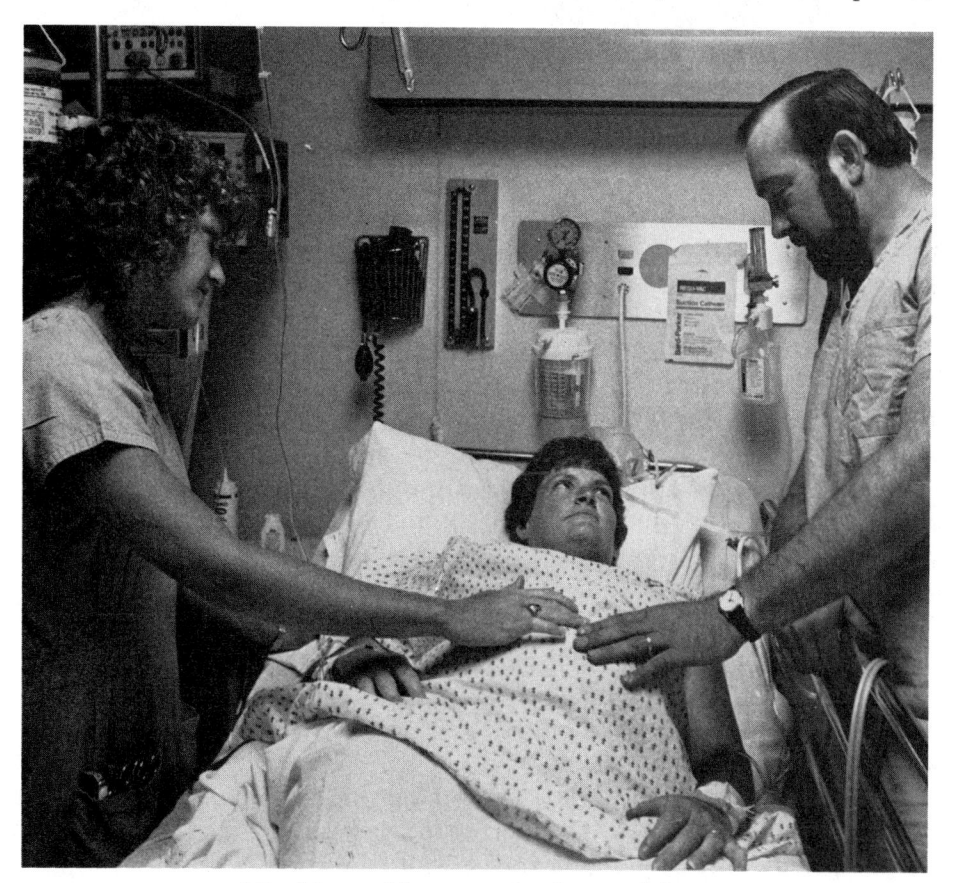

Working with a couple during labor.

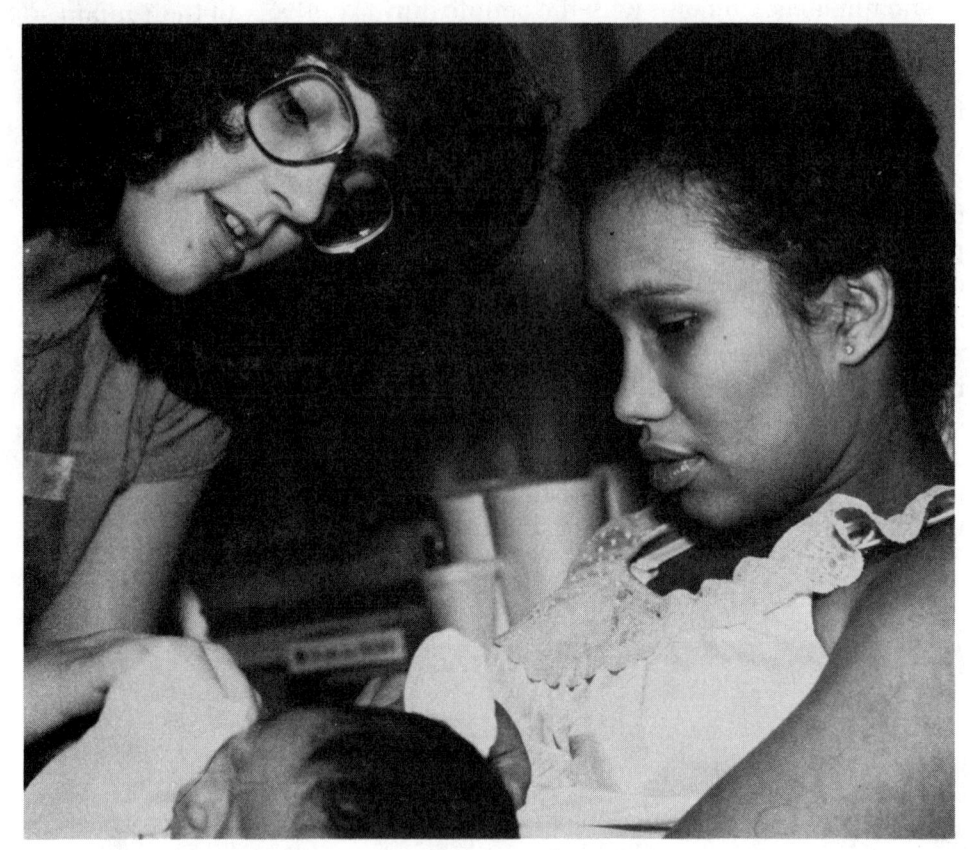

Teaching a new mother about her newborn.

instruments) or she may circulate (the nurse who is not in a sterile gown but who passes things to the scrub team). The circulating nurse is generally responsible for performing the immediate newborn care described previously.

In addition, nurses may be called upon to perform or assist with a number of tests involving pregnant women, such as amniocentesis, a procedure in which amniotic fluid is withdrawn from the woman's uterus, or ultrasonic scanning, which uses sound waves to produce pictures showing where the afterbirth is located, the diameters of the fetus' chest and head, or fetal abnormalities. The nurse can also use fetal monitoring to evaluate changes in fetal heart rate when the fetus moves inside the woman's uterus, and tell how the fetus may respond to the stress of labor.

Care of a woman during labor and delivery requires continuous evaluation of her progress and careful recording on her chart, and on the baby's records during and after delivery. If an emergency occurs, quick decision-making is needed. It is often necessary to work with equipment and machines, making sure they are clean and functioning.

You will be called upon to support women, their husbands, other family members and often physicians who are under stress. As a nurse you will use many technical skills (giving injections, working with monitors, performing or helping with tests), as well as communication and teaching skills.

The most satisfying aspects of the work that nurses mention include sharing the birth of an infant with the couple, helping women feel good about how well they performed in labor, seeing a family happy with their newborn and making it through emergencies successfully. The most frustrating aspects of the work cited by nurses include the recording and paperwork, malfunctioning equipment, emergency situations that end unsuccessfully and caring for women or couples who do not seem to care about or want their newborn.

CHARACTERISTICS IMPORTANT FOR THIS TYPE OF WORK INCLUDE:

- ability to handle stress
- ability to remain calm yet make decisions and act quickly
- ability to commmunicate well
- interest in working with your hands and with equipment

Newborn Intensive Care Unit

A nurse working in the neonatal intensive care unit (NICU) usually begins the shift at 7 A.M., 3 P.M. or 11 P.M. On a typical day the nurse arrives about 6:40 A.M. to change into a hospital scrub suit and get ready for report from the nurse who has taken care of the babies during the past eight hours.

The oncoming nurse is assigned one or two infants and in report finds out all about their conditions, whether they're better or worse, their medications, intravenous fluids or findings, how they're breathing or their ventilator requirements, and what to expect for the day, such as tests. The babies in the unit may have lung problems, need or have had surgery, be premature or have congenital heart problems. Many of the infants weigh less than three pounds. The nurse also finds out if the parents have called or come in and what concerns they are having at this time. The report enables nurses to anticipate and plan for some of the events of the day.

Following report, the nurse must assess each tiny patient's heart rate, respiratory rate, temperature and blood pressure (vital signs) to get baseline evaluations for the day. All of the equipment the babies are on is then checked, to make certain it is working properly.

Throughout the day, every two to four hours, the nurse must recheck the infant's vital signs and equipment, give medications and feedings, and do any treatments required in the infant's care. This might include suctioning the nose and throat or endotracheal tube, changing surgical dressings, drawing blood, changing an intravenous line and fluids, plus providing a lot of tender loving care to the sick babies.

The nurse may also have to prepare for a new admission, go to the delivery room and assist with a premature delivery, or receive a baby who was transported from another hospital. It may be a planned admission but usually it's not.

When the parents of the patients visit, the NICU nurse talks with them and answers their questions. The nurse may set up conferences with physicians for the parents, teach them about their baby's care and encourage them to touch and hold their baby whenever possible. If a baby is nearing the time of discharge, the nurse helps parents learn how to take care of their baby at home and helps them feed, bathe, dress and comfort him.

Sometimes babies do die. The nurse caring for a dying baby must do as much as possible to keep the infant comfortable and also to support family members if they are present.

At the end of the day the nurse gives report to the nurse(s) who will be caring for the same infants for the next eight hours. The nurse ending the shift informs them of what went on during the day and documents in writing what happened so that other members of the health care team (other nurses, physicians, respiratory therapists, pharmacists, social workers) are kept informed round the clock.

Satisfactions identified by nurses working in the neonatal intensive care unit include caring for very sick infants and helping them get well, working with families, learning advanced technical and psychosocial skills, and the excitement that the intensive care atmosphere provides for a variety of experiences.

Frustrations of this type of work include the unpredictability of each day, dealing with death, stress associated with each new situation and stress associated with working with families in crisis.

CHARACTERISTICS IMPORTANT FOR THIS TYPE OF WORK INCLUDE:

- ability to work closely with families
- desire to learn technical skills
- adaptability to various responsibilities throughout a day
- ability to make fast and accurate decisions

Newborn Transport Nursing

The transport nurse's day begins with a phone call from a hospital wanting to transfer a sick baby. The nurse may be on call in the hospital or at home. The call may come at any time of the day or night.

Once the decision to transport the baby is made, the transport team members and the necessary equipment are quickly gathered. It is the transport nurse's responsibility to ensure that all of the equipment is available and in working order. The nurse must anticipate the baby's condition so that extra medications, including oxygen, are taken on the transport. Many smaller hospitals that refer infants do not have supplies of the items carried with the transport team so the team must be self-sufficient and the nurses must know what is there. Preparation time is limited to a maximum of 30 minutes if team members are called in from home and 15 minutes if they are in the hospital.

The team is transported by a specially designed ambulance if the baby is less than 50 miles away. Many transports are done with airplanes or helicopters.

During the trip to the referring hospital, the nurse has time to set up intravenous fluids and warm the incubator. In the ambulance there is generator power to run equipment but in a plane there is not, so the nurse must constantly be aware of how much battery energy the equipment is using so that it can be minimized.

Upon arrival, the nurse assesses the infant and takes vital signs—heart rate, respiratory rate, temperature and blood pressure. Usually the nurse must start an intravenous line and may have to assist with or perform chest tube insertion, and endotracheal intubation to put the baby on a ventilator.

The nurse also talks with the parents about their baby's condition. Usually the nurse takes a picture of the baby to leave with the parents, gives them the phone number of the unit where their baby will be and explains such policies as visitation and calling in.

When the baby's vital signs are stabilized within normal limits, the trip back begins. The baby must be as stable as possible because, for example, on the airplane it is very difficult to do procedures with lack of room and turbulence. If an ambulance is used, it can pull off the road, if necessary, while a procedure is performed, such as putting the baby on a ventilator.

During the return trip, the nurse checks the baby's vital signs every 15 minutes to every hour depending on the baby's condition and must regularly check the pressure in the oxygen tank so that it can be changed if necessary.

Upon arrival at the home hospital, the baby is taken directly to the neonatal intensive care unit. The transport nurse gives the report on the baby to the admitting nurse and the family. When the baby is fully admitted, the transport nurse then cleans the incubator and restocks equipment in preparation for the next transport.

Satisfactions cited by nurses in this type of work include experiencing many different situations, since each transport varies, learning how different hospitals care for infants and learning advanced skills.

Frustrations with transport nursing include being on call and being called in the middle of the night, equipment breakdowns and the stress of each transport.

CHARACTERISTICS IMPORTANT FOR THIS TYPE OF WORK INCLUDE:

- ability to make decisions quickly
- self-direction, especially in learning advanced skills
- flexibility
- commitment to a team approach

Outpatient Clinic

Unless the clinic is open during the weekend or extends its hours into the evening, the staff nurse working in a clinic will probably work an eight-hour shift during the day, Monday through Friday. This type of work can be rewarding since nurses usually see the same patients over a prolonged period of time and this gives a satisfying continuity

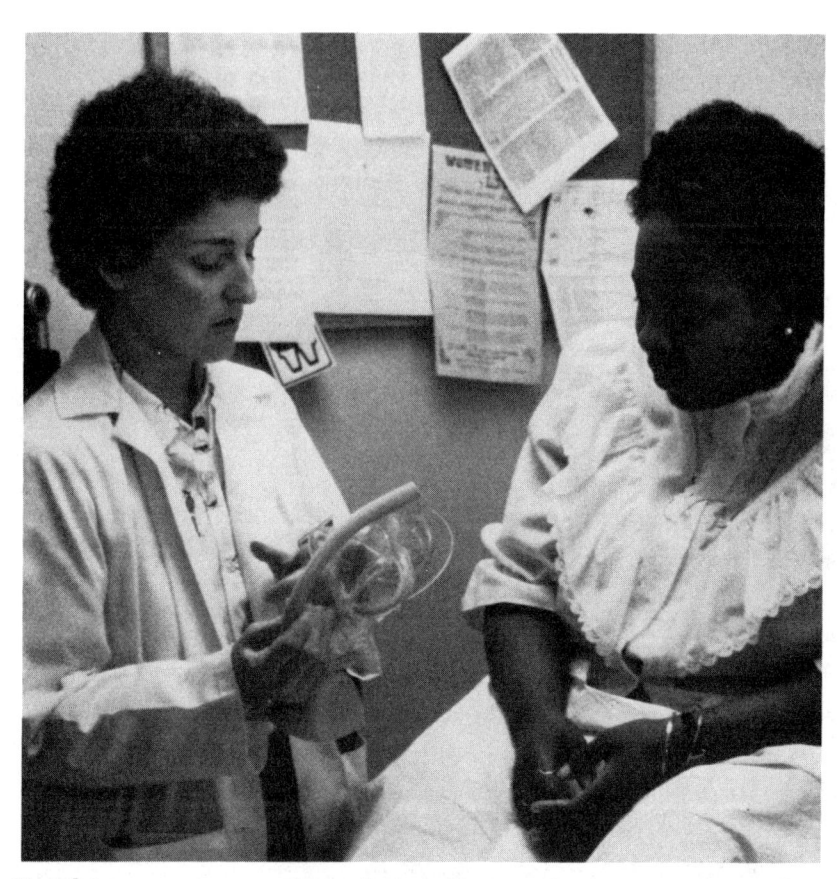

Teaching a woman about her anatomy during a visit to the outpatient department.

to care. In addition, it provides an opportunity to evaluate the outcomes of teaching and other strategies used to bring about patient improvement.

The nurse's day might begin by helping get the clinic ready for the patients by making sure all of the equipment and supplies that will be needed during the day are on hand. The nurse performs selected portions of physical examinations on patients, taking height, weight, temperature, pulse, respiration, blood pressure, and perhaps evaluating lung sounds. If it is a clinic for pregnant women the nurse may listen for and evaluate fetal heart sounds, evaluate how far the uterus has enlarged since the woman's last visit, test urine specimens for sugar and protein, or perform a pregnancy test from the urine. The portion of the physical examination the nurse performs will depend a great deal on the type of clinic, the age and type of patients attending, the requirements of the position and the nurse's own skills. As noted in Chapter 3, some clinics are managed by nurses who consult with the physician only when they encounter problems beyond their expertise, or if they need to write prescriptions for certain drugs beyond those they are permitted to prescribe according to routine backup physician orders.

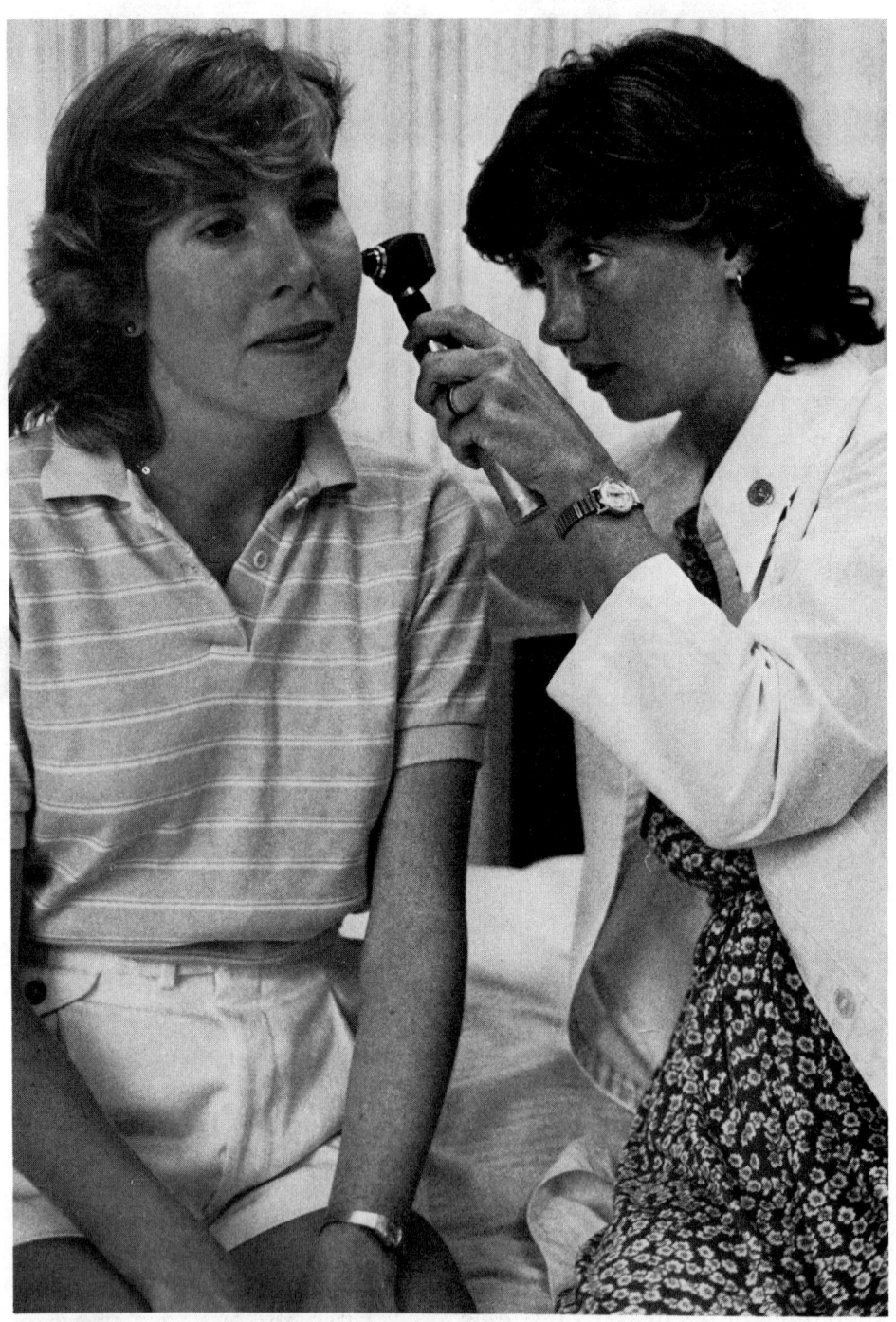

Nurses in outpatient clinics work with a variety of problems.

Hospitals

The staff nurse may evaluate the patient's progress during the period since the last clinic visit. How has he been functioning at home and at work? Have there been any further signs or symptoms of his condition? The nurse checks the patient's diet and response to any medications that were ordered. The clinic nurse teaches individual patients or groups of patients, helping them learn more about their conditions, medications and how to cope with their disorders. Patients may be referred to other members of the health team for special problems. For example, the social worker might be most helpful in finding housing on a lower floor for a man with a severe heart condition. The nutritionist is invaluable in assisting diabetics with their diets.

During the course of the day, part of the staff nurse's effort is directed toward maintaining the flow of patients into and out of examining rooms so that everyone is seen in a reasonable time period. While some clinics may operate on a first come, first seen basis, most use an appointment system.

In addition to performing portions of the physical examination, taking histories, teaching and referring patients to other team members, the nurse may be involved with evaluations or review conferences in which the progress and problems of patients are determined by the health team.

Clinic nurses have identified some of the most satisfying aspects of this work as being the good work schedule and hours, having holidays off and seeing the same patients over a period of months or even years. The most frustrating aspects of the position have been identified as the lack of time to spend with individual patients, physicians arriving late to see patients and patients not keeping their clinic appointments.

CHARACTERISTICS IMPORTANT FOR THIS TYPE OF WORK INCLUDE:

- interest in teaching
- interest in communicating with people
- capacity to remain unfrustrated by routine

Other Staff Nursing Positions

In addition to the staff nurse positions described previously, there are many other services found in hospital settings that offer a variety of chances to use special skills.

Infection Control

Nurses in infection control are responsible for monitoring the hospital for infections and reporting their findings to various decision-making groups. They conduct classes for hospital personnel on how to control the spread of infections among patients and staff. This is a very important role because many patients in hospitals are receiving treatment drugs that reduce their resistance to disease. Therefore, these nurses must check constantly to determine which infections occurred prior to a patient's admission and those that might have been acquired during hospitalization.

Burn Units

Nurses in burn units remain with their patients almost constantly during their shifts. The condition of severely burned patients is precarious. Therefore, they must be carefully observed at all times for complications that might result in sudden death. Nurses remain with these patients over the long period of time it takes them to go from the postburn stage, through skin grafting and rehabilitation.

Pediatric Units

These units specialize in the care of children of all ages who have a variety of chronic illnesses, such as heart disease, asthma and diabetes. There are also those who need surgery, such as appendectomies and repairs of hernias and broken limbs, and children who need a variety of tests. Nurses not only work with the youngsters but also teach parents about normal growth and development as well as child safety and care of the child's particular condition. Some pediatric units are developed for and will admit adolescents.

Intensive Care Units

Nurses in these units provide lifesaving and life sustaining care to critically or severely ill patients in highly specialized units. Very often the nurses must intervene on their own, using standing physican orders,

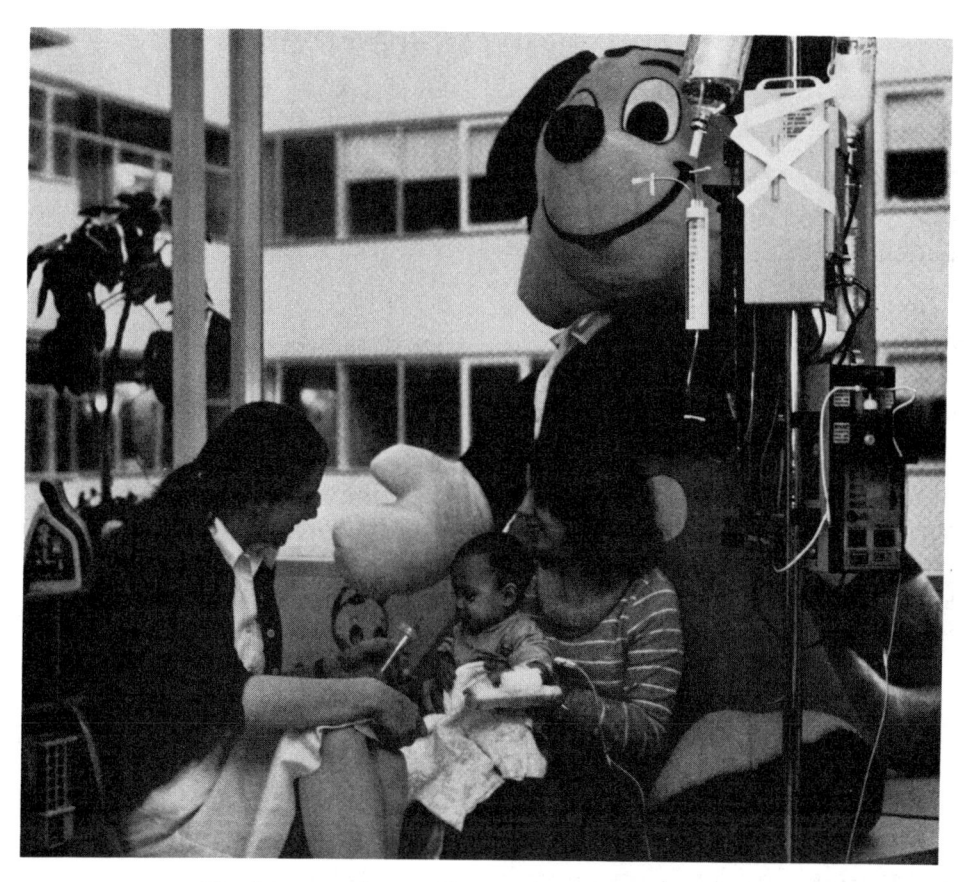

Working with an ill child in a pediatric unit.

if the patient's condition changes suddenly. These units usually contain the latest advances in medical technology. Large hospitals or health centers may have cardiac, surgical, medical, respiratory, pediatric and newborn intensive care units.

Medical Units

Nurses in these units care for adult men and women who have long-term diseases, such as asthma, emphysema, heart problems, high blood pressure, ulcers and diabetes. Since these patients are readmitted for repeated bouts of their disease, nurses may see these same patients over a number of years. Other patients in these units may be in the hospital for tests and diagnosis of a health problem. In some large hospitals there may be separate medical units for patients with cardiac, respiratory and neurologic disorders.

Reseach Units

Some large medical centers have specific units for children or adults with very rare conditions. Nurses in these units participate in research that is aimed at finding out the cause, course, treatment and care of patients with these unusual disorders.

Gynecological Units

Nurses in these units care for women with reproductive problems. Some may have vaginal infections or need minor or major surgery to correct their reproductive organs. Nurses are responsible for care of the women before and after surgery. They may assist with diagnostic tests and treatments, teach breast self-examination, hygienic care and contraceptive practice.

Orthopedic Units

Nurses in these units care for patients with broken or diseased bones and muscle disorders. Very often these patients have body or limb casts and are in the units for prolonged periods of time.

EENT Units

Patients are admitted to these services who have ailments of their eyes, ears, nose or throat. Some patients are totally or partially blind and need cataracts removed or other eye surgery. Some require surgery on their nasal passages or throats due to small growths that must be removed. Still others require middle-ear surgery to restore their hearing or repair their eardrums. Many patients on these units are elderly.

Transplant Units

Patients in these units are usually stressed physically and emotionally. Nurses working with them need to be able to provide excellent physical care as well as emotionally supportive care to both the patients and their families.

Oncology Units

Patients in these units have a variety of types of cancer. They also represent a variety of ages. Because the patients return repeatedly for courses of therapy, nurses become close to the patients and their families.

Detoxification Units

Patients are admitted to these units for resolution of drug or alcohol abuse. Nurses who work in these units need an excellent background in handling people who are emotionally dependent and who display a great deal of manipulative behavior. Caring for these patients is challenging and can be emotionally draining.

Private Duty Nursing

In private duty nursing the nurse cares for one patient for the day, evening or night shift for as long as the patient employs the nurse. Sometimes patients may have private duty nurses for each of the three shifts for the duration of the very serious stage of their illness. These nurses are hired by the patient or the patient's family and are paid directly by them.

Temporary Agency Nursing

When working for a medical pool or temporary agency, nurses are informed of available jobs in local hospitals or health agencies that need nurses for a specific shift, day, week or longer. The nurses then decide what shifts they will work, which hospital or agency they will work in, which position they will take and how many days they will work. Many nurses have chosen to work with these agencies because they can control their own schedules. The pay per shift is also generally higher than that of staff nurses working permanently in the same hospitals.

Types of Nursing Care Delivery

Primary Nursing

Nurses who deliver primary nursing provide total nursing care for a small number of patients (perhaps four to six) from the time of patients' admission to their discharge or transfer to another unit. For patients, primary nursing means that one nurse is responsible for their care 24 hours a day. That nurse works with the patient, physician, social worker and other departments to plan and coordinate the patient's total care. For the nurses, primary nursing restores the authority for decisions on nursing care back where it belongs—with the nurse responsible for the patient's care. Physicians and other health team members seek out the primary nurse instead of the head nurse for updates on the patient's status and for collaboration in treatment decisions. If a patient's treatment schedules are unclear or if there are problems with various departments' ability to deliver services to the patient, the primary nurse may initiate a conference with the physician, social worker, nutritionist or other health team members to resolve the problems. This type of collaboration and system of nursing care delivery has resulted in much improved patient outcomes. Primary nursing is the most recent approach to nursing care delivery.

Team Nursing

In team nursing, professional and nonprofessional personnel work together in teams to plan, provide and evaluate patient care. A nurse on a team may work with other RN's, with licensed practical nurses, nurses' aides and orderlies. Assignment of patients to team members is done by an RN team leader who assigns team members to care for patients whose needs best match the specific members' capabilities. Aides and orderlies may be assigned to care for less ill patients. Team members work together to provide individualized and comprehensive patient care. Patient care conferences are held and attended by all team members. During the conferences, team members discuss their patients' health problems, previous medical histories, emotional status and ways of solving patients' problems. The nurse caring for the patient and the other team members develop care plans for each patient assigned to their team.

Unlike primary nursing, patients may have many nurses or aides and orderlies caring for them during the course of their stay or even during one 24-hour day.

Functional Nursing

Functional nursing is a task-oriented care delivery system in which nurses complete various duties or "tasks" for each patient assigned to them. One day a nurse might be in charge of taking all the patients' blood pressures, pulses, temperatures and respirations. Another nurse might be in charge of giving all medications and starting all IV's. Still another nurse might be in charge of all treatments for the unit, such as changing wound dressings and applying sterile warm soaks to various body areas. Less experienced personnel such as nurses' aides might be responsible for changing all the beds and other housekeeping duties. Functional nursing is an older form of nursing care delivery which is no longer held in high esteem because it fragments patient care among a number of professionals and nonprofessionals. No one staff nurse is totally responsible for any patient's care under this system, and patients and nurses are often frustrated by some of the situations that arise.

In-Service Educator

If you enjoy teaching, helping people develop in their careers and working with patients in the hospital, a position in in-service education may be for you. The in-service educator's role often involves helping newly hired nurses become oriented to the hospital and the units in which they will work, and experienced staff nurses to learn new techniques, or use of new equipment. The educator also serves on hospital committees, carries out educational programs and helps to evaluate nurses' skills. This position demands an excellent and practical grasp of clinical situations. Of equal importance is staying on top of new developments and being able to present them in ways that will help to change in-house practice. The position is usually eight hours a day, Monday through Friday. The starting time for each day may differ according to what the day's schedule involves. Larger hospitals may have a staff of in-service educators, some of whom work during the evening or night shifts. In smaller hospitals, the educator's schedule may vary in order to be pres-

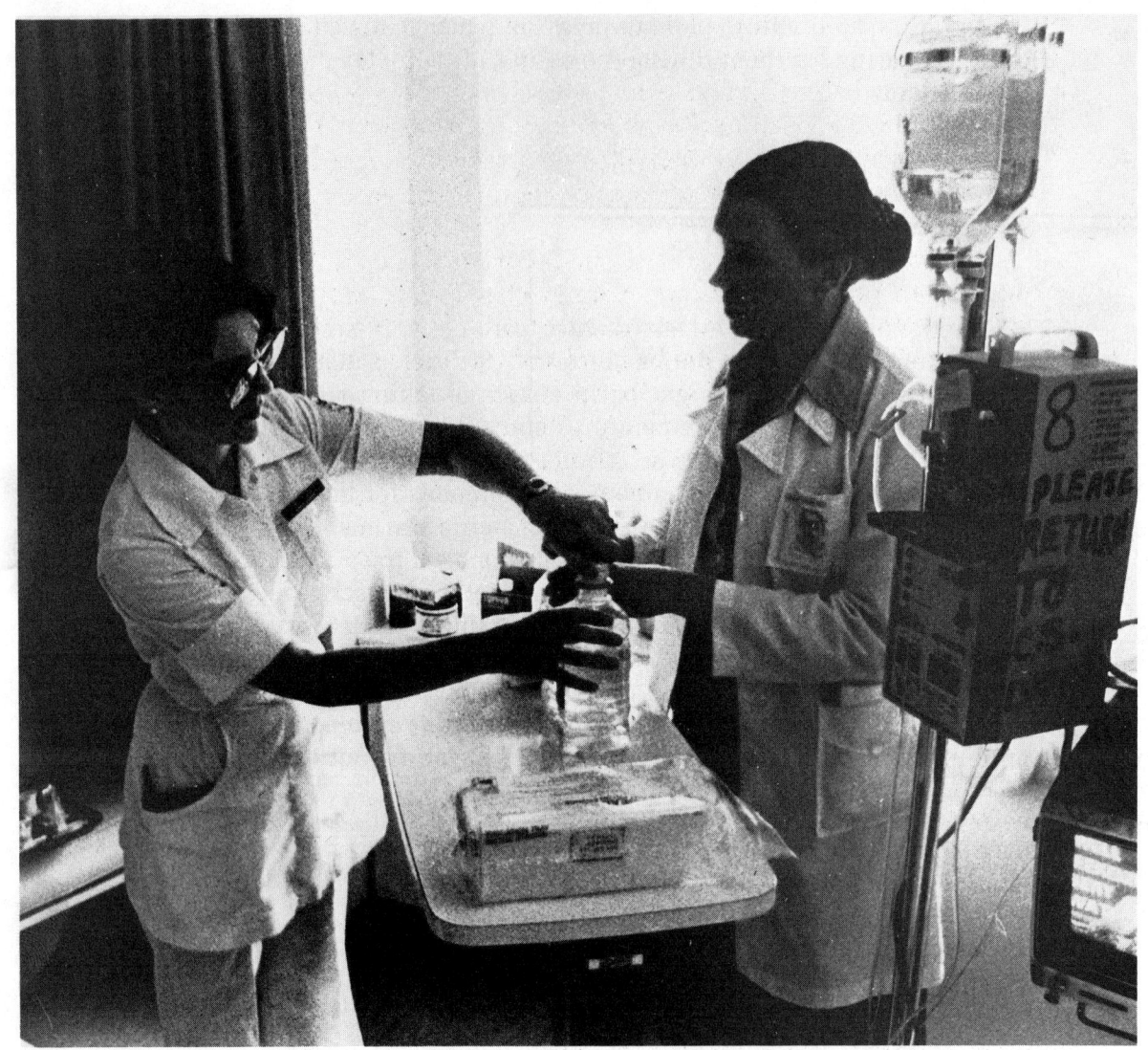

In-service educator working with a new staff nurse.

ent during part of the evening shift. On other days it may be necessary to come in early to spend time with nurses who work the night shift.

An in-service educator's day often begins with a presentation to nurses on the night shift who are nearing the end of their working hours. The topic may be related to patient care—(perhaps an improved way of delivering nursing care), how to work more effectively with families or a new procedure, technique, or piece of equipment the nurses will be using.

Following the morning presentation, in-service educators often make rounds on the patient care units they are assigned to. During these rounds, they talk with the head nurse, the patients and the staff nurses to determine if any of the nurses need help with a new procedure or with the care of a particularly difficult patient. This time would also be used to identify teaching programs the staff nurses need, or that they feel they need, to improve their nursing care. Following rounds, planned demonstrations of new procedures or equipment in each unit might be given.

A significant part of most in-service educators' time is devoted to the orientation program for newly employed nurses at the hospital. Orientation programs for new nurses range from two to twelve weeks depending upon the size of the hospital and the type of unit in which the nurses will be working. If the turnover rate of new nurses is high, the in-service educator may spend considerable time repeating the orientation program. During the orientation program, the in-service educator may present classes on the diseases, treatments and nursing care found most commonly in the units in which the new staff will work. Other nurses, physicians, nutritionists and people from additional specialty groups may teach some of the classes. Therefore, in-service educators must be familiar with the human resources available in the institution and be able to maintain good working relations with them. Evaluation of the nursing skills of newly hired nurses as they begin working in units is an important part of this job, not only from the point of view of judging the effectiveness of the new nurses but for revising and perfecting the teaching program.

An in-service educator may be responsible for the larger task of planning or conducting in-service education programs for the hospital. These might include programs in cardiopulmonary resuscitation, electrical safety or fire safety. The in-service educator must attend many meetings during the course of the day, such as meetings with the head nurses about patient care and nursing staff issues, or as a member of one or more hospital committees. To keep current, time must be spent meeting with sales representatives from medical supply companies about new equipment and its use. This information is used to develop accurately written procedures on the use of new equipment and effective teaching methods for demonstrations. In addition, memos may need to be written to tell when equipment will be available on the units and a schedule may need to be prepared for demonstrations. Nurse educators may also be charged with revising or introducing new methods of recording procedures, such as intravenous solutions or how much food or fluids patients have taken.

Nurses in in-service education identify the most satisfying aspects of the work to include seeing improvements in the delivery of care to patients, and the feeling that they have helped nurses develop in their skills and in their careers. The most frustrating aspect of the position is that the educator often can only *suggest* changes in patient care since most of these positions carry no authority to enact the suggestions. The head nurse or staff nurse must carry the changes through. Another frustration commonly mentioned is that considerable persuasion may be needed to convince staff that the program offerings are an important part of growing in their jobs.

CHARACTERISTICS IMPORTANT FOR THIS TYPE OF WORK INCLUDE:

- good communication skills
- persuasive negotiating skills
- discrimination
- interest in teaching

The educational requirements for a position as an in-service educator generally range from a bachelor's in nursing to a master's degree. The position also requires experience in nursing practice. A background in teaching is helpful. Salaries for the position are variable depending upon the size and location of the hospital, but are usually comparable to that of a head nurse.

Career Advancement

Nurses in in-service education often advance their careers by pursuing teaching careers in schools of nursing, becoming heads of in-sevice educational departments or by pursuing careers in nursing administrative positons.

Clinical Specialist

A clinical specialist is a nurse who has highly developed knowledge in one area of nursing, for example, pediatrics, psychiatry or school health. This nurse's role often involves teaching, consultation, research and management. The specialist may teach patients and sometimes carry a case load of patients. More often, specialists use their expertise to

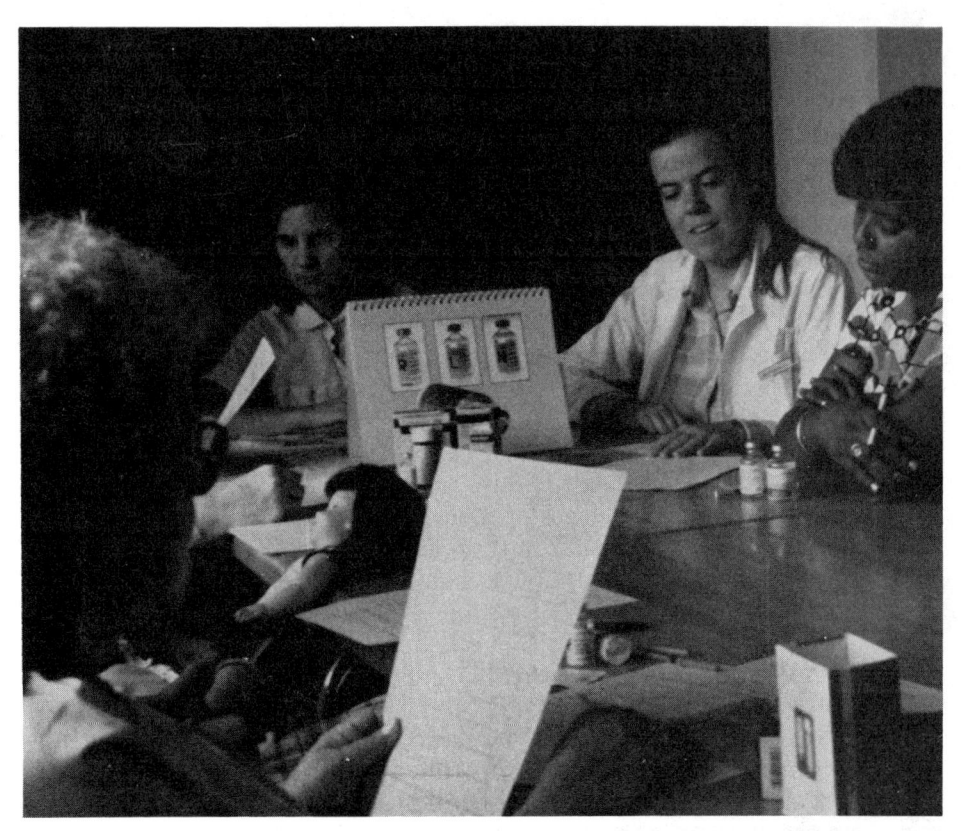

Clinical specialist working with a group of patients.

teach and serve as consultants to staff nurses who are trying to deal with difficult situations or patients whose care is complex. The clinical specialist may also serve as a consultant to community groups involved in health care and to nurses in other hospitals. Many clinical specialists also participate in nursing research and very often identify patient problems that need to be researched in order to improve care. The specialist may be assigned to a particular unit in the hospital or may be available to many units for consultation and assistance.

A psychiatric clinical specialist who works with staff in critical care, dialysis, transplant and cancer units describes her work in the following way:

> The staff on these units work in a very stressful atmosphere. Very often they feel overly responsible for patients and their prognosis. She helps them sort out the sources of stress and gives them support in handling the problems associated with patient care, such as helping a patient die comfortably. This involves examining the limits of a nurse's ability to control the course of a patient's condition.

Following rounds on one unit, she conducts support groups for staff and head nurses on another unit. During the sessions, issues that came up during the week are discussed. They might include how to improve communications among the nurses, between nurses and physicians or nurses and patients, and how to take breaks from a busy unit without feeling guilty. Other topics might be how to handle angry patients, depressed and suicidal patients and patients whose outlook is hopeless. Some time during the week she also conducts staff support groups for the evening and night nurses.

Following the support groups for staff nurses, she attends patient groups. These groups are conducted by patients who meet to share common concerns about their conditions, have questions answered and provide support for one another. Many of the groups are patients with severe heart conditions or those who have advanced stages of cancer. She answers their questions, corrects any misinformation they have and offers family members suggestions on how to help the patients at home.

This clinical specialist works more than 40 hours each week but her hours are flexible. She schedules her time each week according to the hospital schedule and the needs of the nursing staff on the units she covers.

She finds the most satisfying aspects of her work include working with the staff nurses and helping them improve their care and their ability to cope with the demands of work. Helping nurses develop in their roles, realize their potential and enjoy their jobs are very satisfying aspects of her work. Her frustrations center around not having enough time to do all that she feels should be done with patients and staff.

Her day begins with rounds on one of several units to which she provides consultation. For the next two hours she is available to the nursing staff and makes rounds with them to help solve patient care problems.

Another kind of clinical specialist in women's health works with parents of dead or dying newborn infants in conjunction with the attending obstetrician. Expectant parents spend many months looking forward to the birth of their newborns. They plan and dream about how they will look, what they will do and how they will develop. Parents of dead or terminally ill newborns, instead of carrying home a bright-eyed infant, carry home their empty plans and dreams. These clinical specialists help parents go through the grieving process. They talk with the parents about the feelings they can expect—shock or denial, sadness, guilt, depression and anger. They evaluate where a couple is in the grieving process and encourage communication between the two. If the couple have other children the specialist talks about how to explain the loss of the baby to them. Parents need to understand how important it is to have family support during this period, close relatives they can turn to, and perhaps a minister. There are other practical considerations, such as whether the baby is to be baptized and whether a memorial service is to be had. There are other issues to be discussed as well. Do the parents want an autopsy? Do they want to bury the baby or do they wish the hospital to take care of the baby's body? Would they like a photograph or footprints of the infant? If the newborn had physical defects, blood is drawn for genetic studies. If the studies reveal that the baby's death was due to a genetic problem, the parents receive medical counseling for future pregnancies.

If the baby is premature and critically ill, the clinical specialist and the staff nurses encourage the parents to spend time with the infant since this seems to make the grieving process easier. As one clinical specialist notes, "It helps enormously if the baby has been real to the parents." She encourages the parents to see the baby, touch it, name it and note family resemblances. When this occurs, fewer parents return home feeling entirely empty and desolate. The clinical specialist notes that in the case of a stillborn infant, there is no chance for the infant to develop a particular personality or to be perceived as a separate person. In these situations, mothers often feel they have lost a part of their own bodies. The clinical specialist counsels couples to wait six months to a year before attempting another pregnancy, since they often need that much time to grieve for the baby. This clinical specialist's job is personally challenging and invaluable to parents of dead or critically ill newborns.*

CHARACTERISTICS IMPORTANT FOR THIS TYPE OF WORK INCLUDE:

- emotional stability
- flexibility
- a strong ego
- ability to listen
- communication skills
- interest in working with a variety of people
- ability to handle stress

---

*"The Versatile MCP Nurse in Clinical Specialties." *Today*, p. 4, Winter 1981.

The educational requirement for a position as a clinical specialist is a master's degree in nursing. The position also requires experience in nursing practice. Salaries for the position are variable depending upon the size and geographical location of the hospital, but are usually comparable to or better than those of a head nurse.

Career Advancement

Nurses in clinical specialty often advance their careers by pursuing teaching positions in schools of nursing, nursing administration or nursing research.

Head Nurse

Unlike the staff nurse positions described previously, the position of head nurse involves giving little direct care. The head nurse serves in a managerial role and is responsible for the quality of nursing care in the unit. In order to assure the quality of care delivered, negotiations with many individuals in other departments in the hospital—dietary, housekeeping, various laboratories, social service, medicine, pharmacy and medical records—are necessary.

The head nurse's day begins with a report from the night supervisor. The two discuss significant problems in patient care in the unit and in other units within the hospital that are important to be aware of. They also review staffing problems that are anticipated during the day and upcoming evening or night shifts. Following the meeting with the night supervisor, a more detailed report on patients in the unit will be given to the oncoming group of staff nurses by the night nurse who is reporting off.

Following these morning reports, the head nurse assigns patients to specific nurses for care during the day. In some hospitals, this is not necessary because patients are cared for each day by the same nurse until they are discharged (primary nursing). (See "Types of Nursing Care Delivery," pages 48–52.) Any issues specific to the assigned patients are assessed with the nurses who will be caring for them, and rounds may be made with the staff nurses to review a patient's status. If the unit is very busy, the head nurse may help staff nurses with direct care, fitting in where necessary.

Much of the rest of the day will be spent troubleshooting specific

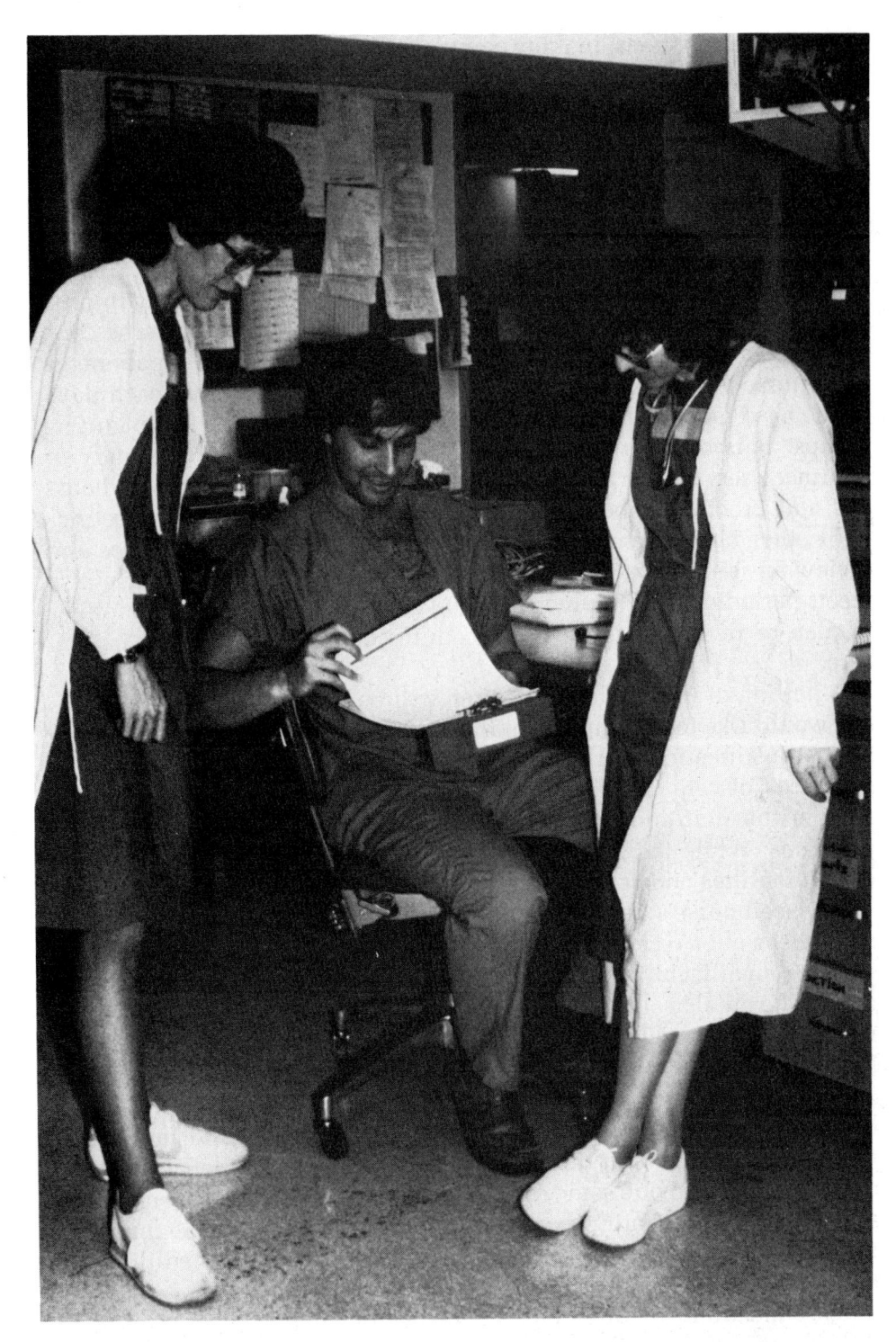

Head nurse and staff nurse consulting with physician.

patient care problems, making rounds with doctors, attending committees, conferences or planning meetings, and completing paperwork.

The troubleshooting role is very important to smooth operation of the unit. It includes such things as trying to straighten out mixups in the scheduling of patients for tests, diets that haven't arrived at the unit for patients, locating supplies or equipment that haven't been delivered to the unit and resolving many emergencies in patient care with the staff nurses and physicians.

A head nurse spends a fair amount of time making rounds with physicians, reviewing patients' progress, treatment plan and nursing care. Since physicians arrive at the unit at different times to see patients, a head nurse may make rounds with several different doctors each day.

The head nurse is also involved with various committee and planning groups. This could include groups working on changes in dietary or pharmacy services, or the public relations department developing booklets and brochures about care or the institution. Periodical meetings with other head nurse groups are important in planning changes and reviewing issues that affect other units as well. The head nurse also meets periodically with physicans and counterparts in other disciplines to plan or review changes in procedures or policies affecting patient care.

A portion of the head nurse's time will be spent developing changes she would like to accomplish in the unit. This might include preparing budget justifications for increased staff, patient teaching programs or standards of care. More time will be spent in evaluating the nursing staff in the unit and identifying and planning for staff development programs. While the head nurse will not present these programs, she often identifies and seeks out the people who will.

The head nurse's day ends much as it begins, sitting with the evening supervisor after receiving a brief report from the staff nurses and reviewing significant problems or issues regarding patients in the unit, and the hospital itself. Following this meeting, a designate or the primary nurses will give a report on the patients to the oncoming shift of nurses. Many head nurses remain in the unit until the night shift gets underway.

Some of the most satisfying aspects of the position as identified by head nurses are helping staff nurses develop their skills and career, and seeing improvements in the delivery of patient care in their units. The opportunity to provide some direct care to patients has also been viewed as a plus. The frustrating aspects of the position are seen as the rapid turnover of nursing staff, not enough staff nurses and scheduling the nurses' time.

The educational requirements for the position of head nurse vary with the size and geographical location of the hospital and may range from a diploma to a master's degree in nursing. Salaries range between $15,000 and $25,000, depending on size of the hospital and area of the country.

Career Advancement

Head nurses often advance their careers by becoming nursing supervisors, assistant directors, directors of nursing or vice presidents of hospitals. (See Figure 2.) Other head nurses may pursue careers by teaching nursing in a school of nursing or in an in-service education department of the hospital.

Examples of Job Hierarchies in Hospitals

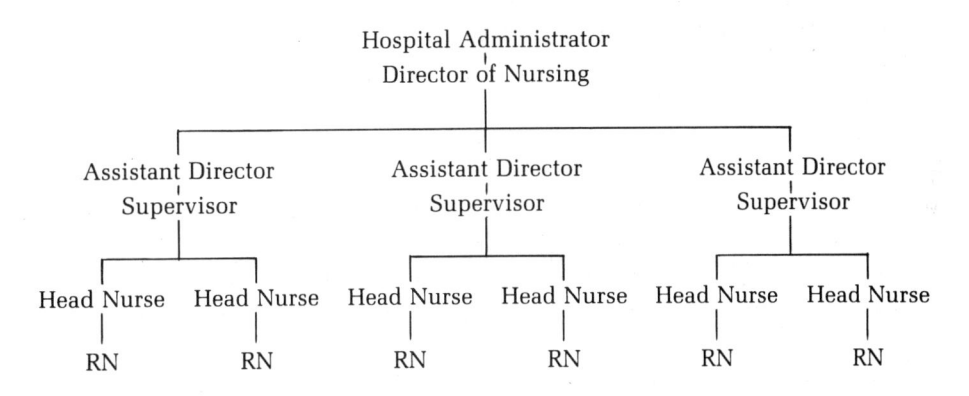

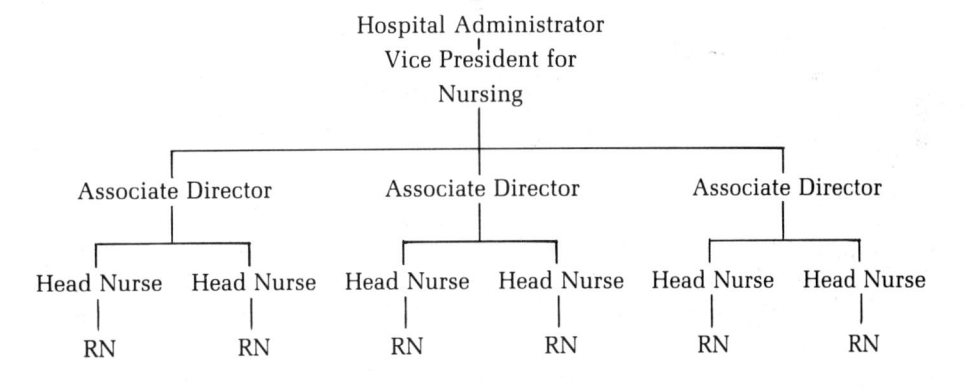

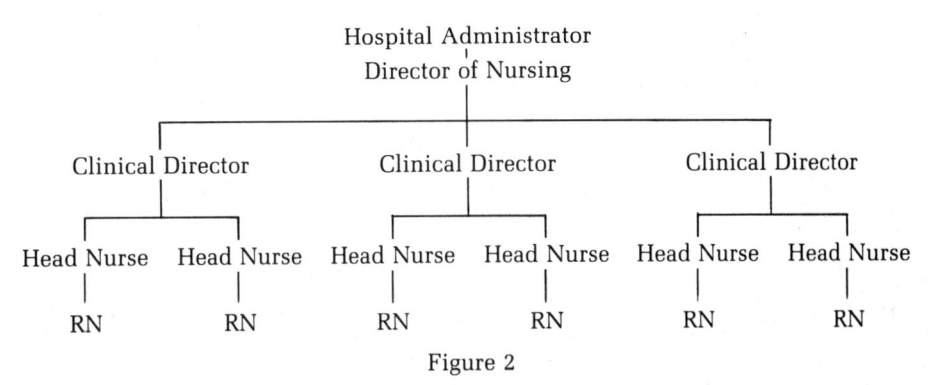

```
                  Hospital Administrator
                   Director of Nursing
         ┌─────────────────┼─────────────────┐
   Assistant Director  Assistant Director  Assistant Director
      Supervisor          Supervisor          Supervisor
     ┌─────┴─────┐      ┌─────┴─────┐      ┌─────┴─────┐
  Head Nurse  Head Nurse  Head Nurse Head Nurse Head Nurse Head Nurse
     │          │          │          │          │          │
     RN         RN         RN         RN         RN         RN


                  Hospital Administrator
                   Vice President for
                        Nursing
         ┌─────────────────┼─────────────────┐
   Associate Director  Associate Director  Associate Director
     ┌─────┴─────┐      ┌─────┴─────┐      ┌─────┴─────┐
  Head Nurse  Head Nurse  Head Nurse Head Nurse Head Nurse Head Nurse
     │          │          │          │          │          │
     RN         RN         RN         RN         RN         RN


                  Hospital Administrator
                   Director of Nursing
         ┌─────────────────┼─────────────────┐
    Clinical Director   Clinical Director   Clinical Director
     ┌─────┴─────┐      ┌─────┴─────┐      ┌─────┴─────┐
  Head Nurse  Head Nurse  Head Nurse Head Nurse Head Nurse Head Nurse
     │          │          │          │          │          │
     RN         RN         RN         RN         RN         RN
```

Figure 2

CHARACTERISTICS IMPORTANT FOR THIS TYPE OF WORK INCLUDE:

- assertiveness
- persistence
- interest in helping other people develop their careers
- ability to work with various people of varying backgrounds, personalities and status
- ability to plan and organize

Assistant Director

The position of assistant director of nursing is an administrative one in which the nurse is responsible for the management of care in one or more portions of the hospital. Although there are variations depending upon the institutional structure, the general responsibilities are for the budget and overall fiscal management of a section, and for staffing. In small hospitals, assistant directors may hire and fire all nursing staff assigned to their section, although in large hospitals some of this task may be delegated to head nurses. Even so, assistant directors may still be involved in firing staff when head nurses feel the need for assistance in this matter.

Assistant directors are responsible for the long range planning in a section of a hospital. In carrying out this work they meet often with their counterparts in the hospital administration and with other nursing assistant directors. Very often the heads or assistant directors of other departments, such as social service, pharmacy, and public relations, must be consulted. The position requires knowledge of organizations, organizational survival and power games, ability to work with other people, and skill in negotiation, compromise and management.

An assistant director's day might begin with the night supervisor to find out any special patient care or other problems in the units or in the hospital in general. The next move might be going through the mail and organizing what must be accomplished that day. The assistant director might then make rounds on one or more units in the hospital before beginning scheduled meetings. Attending or chairing meetings of all kinds is a significant part of this position.

Assistant directors meet at least once a week with the director of nursing about what is going on in the units and to discuss any new policies, procedures, and patient care or staffing issues. Once a year, the assistant director shares with the nursing director the long range plans and objectives that have been developed for the units, and seeks input and approval, prior to having them shared and approved by other hospital groups.

In addition to meetings with the director of nursing, the assistant director meets with other assistant directors approximately once a month for updates on planning or issues that affect each of them at the departmental level. This might include introducing a new type of nursing care delivery or anticipated changes in staffing ratios. Assistant directors also meet with the medical staffs of their units to plan or review long range plans for their division, such as the opening of a new unit or changing the medication distribution system. The assistant directors participate on hospital committees that are responsible for such things as infectious disease control, patient care, critical care, affirmative action and continuing education. They also meet with the unit head nurses to resolve problems they might be encountering and to help them with short-range plans for their unit, such as developing patient teaching programs or in-service programs for their staff.

Another part of the assistant director's day is spent handling problems. These might include complaints from patients, physicians or other hospital services. There is also the work of identifying or developing ways to implement new policies or procedures in the units, responding to correspondence and other types of paperwork. At the end of the day, the assistant director meets with the evening supervisor regarding any patient care, staffing or other problems that might arise during the evening and night shifts.

Assistant directors of nursing have identified some of the most satisfactory aspects of the position as seeing the nursing staff develop in their skills and career, and watching programs to improve care develop and succeed. The most frustrating aspects have been identified as staffing and scheduling problems and the interruptions of program planning that occur as a result.

Depending upon the size and location of the hospital, the educational requirements for the positions vary from a diploma in nursing to a doctoral degree. The salary range is also variable, ranging between $15,000 to $35,000 a year.

CHARACTERISTICS IMPORTANT FOR THIS TYPE OF WORK INCLUDE:

- interest in organizations and organizational behavior
- interest in developing others
- ability to plan and organize

- ability to make decisions
- ability to negotiate and compromise on issues
- a strong nursing identity

Director of Nursing or Chief Nurse Executive

The chief nurse executive is responsible for the nursing department and manages that department so that it contributes to the overall goals of the institution. The nurse at this level is obligated to be a spokesperson for nursing, providing leadership and vision in nursing's development and advancement. Directors of nursing spend much time collaborating with other executives in the hospital so that clear, reasoned decisions about health care services and priorities can be determined. They are also responsible for providing input into community and government decisions that set priorities in meeting the health care needs of the country, developing or restructuring the health care delivery system, changing or creating new health care workers' roles and producing changes which influence the nurse's role. In an administrative role, the nurse executive directs the nursing staff in providing quality nursing care, facilitates nursing research and encourages the use of research and activities which further the clinical practice of nurses.

Some of the responsibilities of this position include:

- participating with top hospital management in decision making, including setting financial and organizational goals
- collaborating with other department heads and administrators in establishing programs and carrying out committee work
- determining the objectives and standards of nursing care within the hospital, and monitoring the quality of nursing care given in the hospital
- structuring the positions within the nursing department and describing who reports to whom
- establishing job descriptions for the positions
- establishing nursing committees
- developing reports on programs, the quality of care, new directions that should be taken by the department, etc.

- planning for staffing the hospital with an adequate number of nurses
- determining the budget for nursing personnel and equipment and supplies
- planning for keeping the nursing staff's knowledge current through in-service programs, encouraging staff to continue their education toward further degrees or through programs of continuing education
- encouraging research that improves patient care
- relating to community and government agencies engaged in studying or making decisions regarding health care
- providing leadership in professional nursing and health care organizations*

For Further Information

Write:

American Nurses Association
2420 Pershing Road
Kansas City, MO 64108

ANA Divisions:

- Gerontological Nursing Practice
- Maternal Child Health Nursing Practice
- Medical-Surgical Nursing Practice
- Psychiatric Mental Health Nursing

American Association of Critical Care Nurses
P.O. Box C-19528
Irvine, CA 92713

---

*"Roles, Responsibilities, and Qualifications for Nurse Administrators." *American Nurses Association*, Publication No. N5–23, 1978.

American Association of Neurosurgical Nurses
625 North Michigan Avenue
Chicago, IL 60611

Association of Operating Room Nurses
10170 East Mississippi Avenue
Denver, CO 80231

Association for Practitioners in Infection Control
23341 North Milwaukee Avenue
Half Day, IL 60069

Emergency Department Nurses Association
666 North Lake Shore Drive
Suite 1131
Chicago, IL 60611

National Association of Orthopedic Nurses, Inc.
Box 56
North Woodbury Road
Pitman, NJ 08071

Nurses Association of the American College
of Obstetricians and Gynecologists
600 Maryland Avenue, S.W.
Suite 200 East
Washington, DC 20024

Oncology Nursing Society
701 Washington Road
Pittsburgh, PA 15228

Read:

Ahmed, M. "Taking Charge of a Change in Hospital Nursing Practice." *American Journal of Nursing* 81:541, 1981.

Burns, L. "Ambulatory Surgery Growing at a Rapid Pace." *AORN Journal* 35:260, 1982.

Cason, C. and Beck, C. "Clinical Nurse Specialist Role Development." *Nursing and Health Care* 3:25, 1982.

Continuing Education in Nursing: An Overview.
   American Nurses Association
   Publication No. COE–10

Harris, A. "HUP Nurse Monitors Intensive Care Ward." *Daily Pennsylvanian*, Philadelphia, April 8, 1982.

Infection Control.
   National League for Nursing
   Publication No. 20-1582

Mullner, R.; Byrne, C.; and Whitehead, S. "Hospital Vacancies." *American Journal of Nursing* 82:592, 1982.

The Role of the Director of Nursing Service.
   National League for Nursing
   Publication No. 20-1646

3.

Independent and Joint Practices

If you would like to have your own case load of patients for whom you perform physical examinations, manage minor illnesses, deliver babies and do teaching and counseling, then a career as an independent nurse practitioner or as a nurse in joint practice with a physician may be for you. This is a rapidly increasing area in nursing both in the number of nurses practicing in it and in the number of nursing specialty areas developing within it. Some of the areas include:

- Pediatric Nurse Practitioner or Clinician
- Certified Nurse Midwife
- Family Nurse Practitioner or Clinician
- Adult Nurse Practitioner or Clinician
- Obstetric and Gynecologic Nurse Practitioner or Clinician
- Certified Registered Nurse Anesthetist
- Family Planning Nurse Practitioner
- Emergency Room Nurse Practitioner
- Neonatal Nurse Practitioner
- School Nurse Practitioner or Clinician
- Gerontologic Nurse Practitioner or Clinician

These independent or joint practice positions require people who enjoy making their own decisions, who are self-directed and who are comfortable functioning autonomously. Nurses in these positions need to be able to work closely and harmoniously with other members of the health care team in sharing responsibility for different aspects of patient care. It is also important to be able to negotiate one's own roles and responsibilities with those of other team members.

These positions are not for the beginning nurse, but rather for those who have had several years of experience and additional educational background. An individual must first become a registered nurse and then seek further preparation in a master's degree or certificate program in nursing. The educational programs for certification as a nurse practitioner range from three to twelve months. Emphasis is placed on practice skills. Upon completion of the program nurses receive a certificate. A nurse clinician program at the master's level ranges in length from one to two years and may incorporate the same skills as a certificate program, but provides a broader educational base that allows greater upward career mobility. Courses such as group dynamics, economics or finance, research, advanced preparation in nursing management and the basic sciences are examples of the courses offered.

Following either type of educational preparation, there is often an examination at the state level to obtain licensure as a nurse practitioner or as a nurse midwife. A nurse midwife must also take a national examination given by the American College of Nurse Midwives.

Getting set up in collaborative or joint practice with one or more physicians may occur in conjunction with grants provided by private foundations interested in this type of approach to health care. Many times physicians seek nurses to join them in their practice because nurses can provide comprehensive care to clients with less complicated problems. This allows physicians to devote their time to clients with complicated clinical problems. Physicians often look for nurse colleagues through educational programs. More often, however, nurses seeking positions send their resumes and a description of the job they want to clinics, hospitals, industries, schools and public health agencies. They also keep a close watch on advertisements in professional magazines and in national newspapers.

Establishing an independent practice requires investment money for office space and equipment, and perhaps an additional full or part-time position when beginning. You can advertise your services through nurse colleagues, local professional organizations, family and friends. Many independent nurse practitioners have found that satisfied patients are the most effective advertisers. Except in states that allow direct reimbursement to nurses from private insurance policies, the nurse's fee comes directly from the patient.

Salaries from joint or collaborative practices vary depending upon the section of the country, the nurse's educational level and experience, whether the nurse is salaried by the physician or whether the nurse receives a percentage of the income of the total practice. Salaries generally range from $15,000 to $30,000 or more.

Educational Preparation for an Expanded Practice Role in Nursing

Registered Nurse

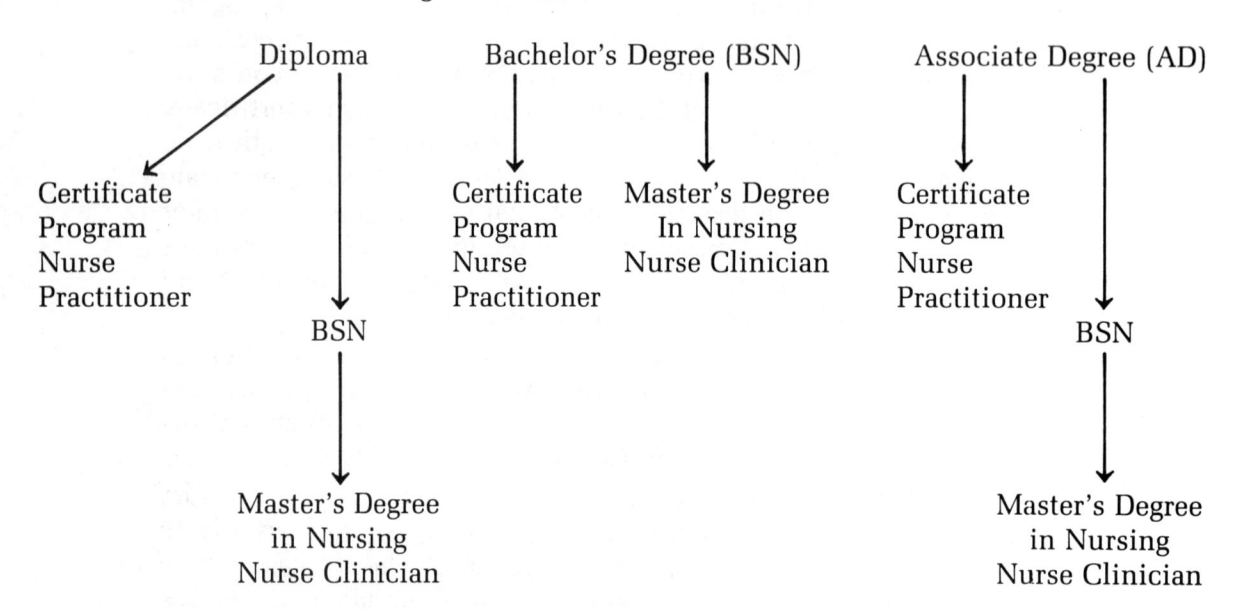

Diploma	Bachelor's Degree (BSN)	Associate Degree (AD)

Certificate Program Nurse Practitioner (from Diploma)

BSN → Master's Degree in Nursing Nurse Clinician (from Diploma)

Certificate Program Nurse Practitioner (from BSN)

Master's Degree In Nursing Nurse Clinician (from BSN)

Certificate Program Nurse Practitioner (from AD)

BSN → Master's Degree in Nursing Nurse Clinician (from AD)

Figure 3

Adult Nurse Clinician

Patricia Hynan, a master's prepared nurse, is representative of adult nurse clinicians in joint practice with a physician. Their office is located in an apartment house for the elderly. Both of them maintain their own case load of patients, referring patients to each other as needed. The twenty dollar fee is the same whether patients see the nurse or the doctor. Patricia's case load of patients includes only elderly adults. Many of her patients are chronically ill with diabetes, high blood pressure or arthritis. Her patients come to her for physical examinations, checkups or when they are having problems with their disease or medications. She evaluates how stable their condition is and teaches them how to deal with problems created by chronic illness. She also gives instruction about the medications they are taking, what side effects may occur and how to combat some of these, and when to contact her if other symptoms should occur. Pat also counsels clients as they try to adjust their lifestyle in response to limitations created by their physical condition. As a sideline, she writes articles for a small newspaper focused on how to stay healthy.

Pat likes her work. She enjoys working with people individually and having them share their concerns with her. She has the time to listen and is able to teach and counsel her clients so that it makes a difference in their ability to get well or stay well. She also appreciates seeing them leave her office satisfied with the care they receive.

Family Nurse Clinician

Satisfied clients are one of the reasons Carmen Ramirez, a master's prepared family nurse clinician, was drawn to specialty nursing practice. She is in practice with two other nurse practitioners and eight physicians. Carmen says that much of the satisfaction she feels comes from helping clients make decisions about their own health. She enjoys watching them adopt more healthy lifestyles and become better able to care for themselves effectively. Carmen also finds working with nurse practitioners and physicians as colleagues a rewarding part of her job.

Carmen has her own patient case load as do the other nurse clinicians and physicians in the joint practice. The group is located in a clinical setting of a major urban teaching hospital. Carmen's case load includes elderly people with chronic illnesses, as well as teenagers and young adults. Her patients are often referred to her by physicians because the patients need extensive health teaching and counseling about their illnesses or changes they need to make in their lives if they are to remain healthy. In addition to teaching and counseling about specific diseases, Carmen works to help people learn how to lose weight, stop smoking and cope with stress and tension. She also does routine physical examinations and monitors patients' drugs and their side effects. Carmen, like Patricia, teaches patients about their drugs, what to expect, and adjusts the doses of their medications as needed. She also teaches patients how to test their blood and urine for levels of sugar and other substances. Most of Carmen's patients are not sick enough to require hospitalization, but their state of health is such that they need to be seen routinely to ensure health maintenance.

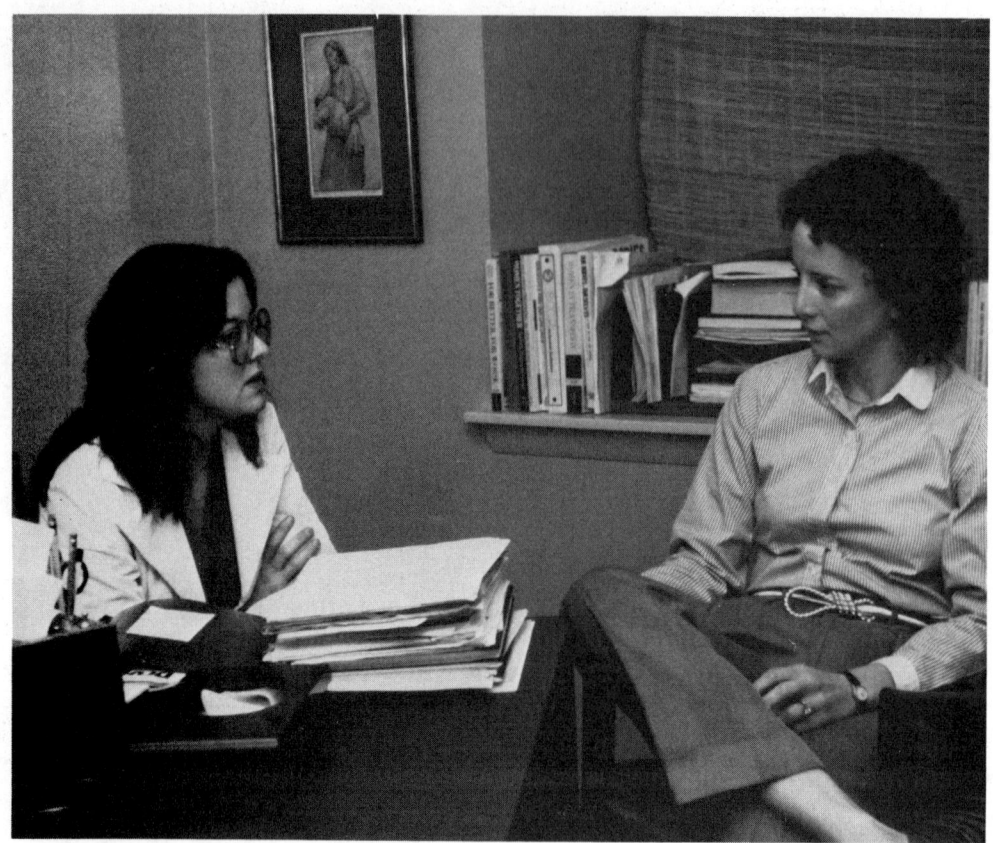

Teaching and counseling are an important part of the nurse's role.

Certified Nurse Midwife

Janet Bolton, a master's prepared nurse, is also a certified nurse midwife in a group practice with two physicians. The physicians and Janet each have their own case load of patients. Janet currently works out of two offices in different locations in a large city. By the end of her first three months of practice, her case load numbered 100 patients with 16 of them enrolled in prenatal care.

As a certified nurse midwife, Janet provides patients who have normal pregnancies with prenatal care, delivers their babies and cares for the mothers after delivery. Many midwives also provide care for infants during their first year of life. Although Janet does not do this, she cares for women who have common gynecological problems, provides contraceptive counseling, prescribes oral contraceptives, fits women with dia-

Independent and Joint Practices 71

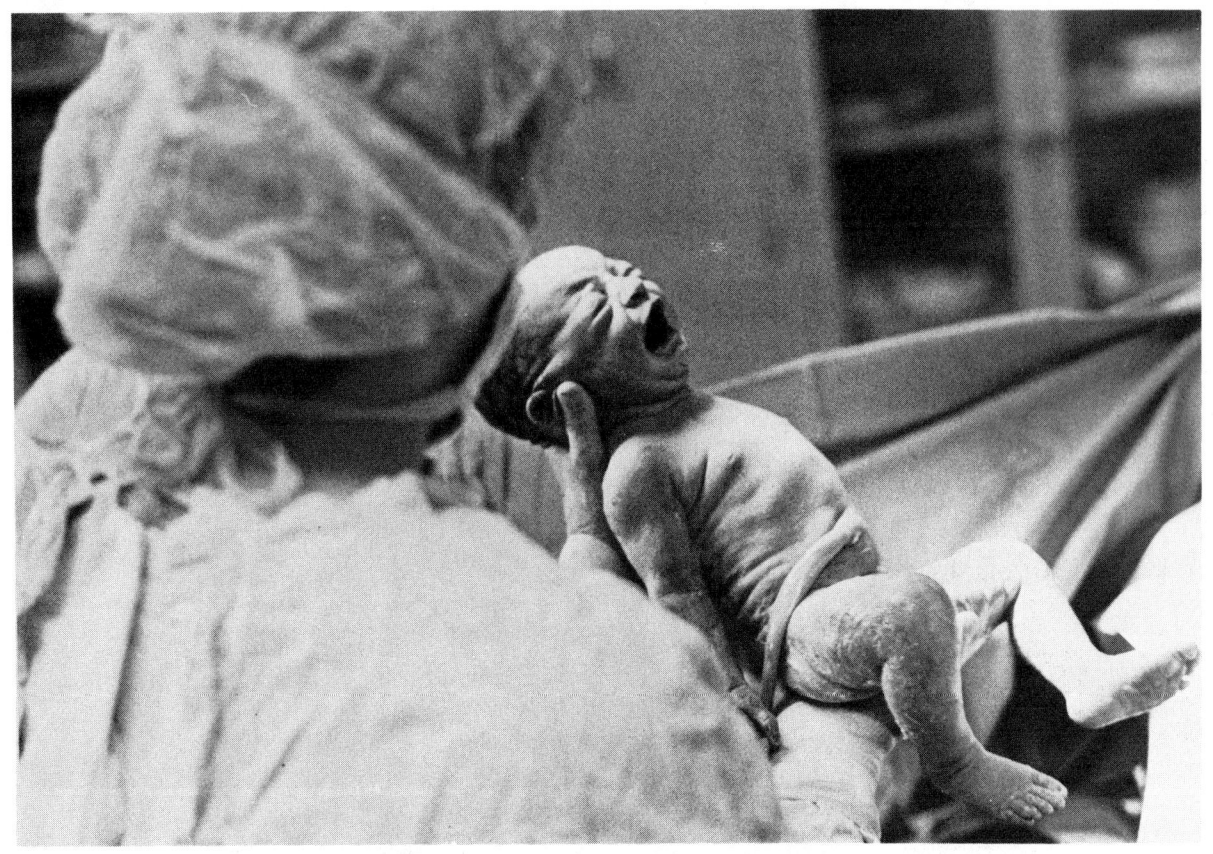

Nurse midwife delivers newborn.

phragms and intrauterine devices (IUD), and teaches couples how to use condoms, foams and natural methods of contraception. Janet also counsels couples on conception. For example, she might advise a woman who has been using an IUD to avoid trying to become pregnant until she has had one or more normal menstrual cycles without the IUD. Irregular menstrual cycles with IUD use are a common cause of miscarriages after IUD removal. Janet also does sexual counseling.

Janet loves her work. She comments that experiencing a birth with a family is one of the most privileged experiences in which one may participate. She feels that becoming intimately involved with a family throughout a pregnancy and helping them through the period of delivery provides an elation that she has encountered in no other career experience. Janet also says she enjoys the independent decision-making and functioning that midwifery practice can provide. She also notes that major frustrations center around state laws which regulate midwifery practice.

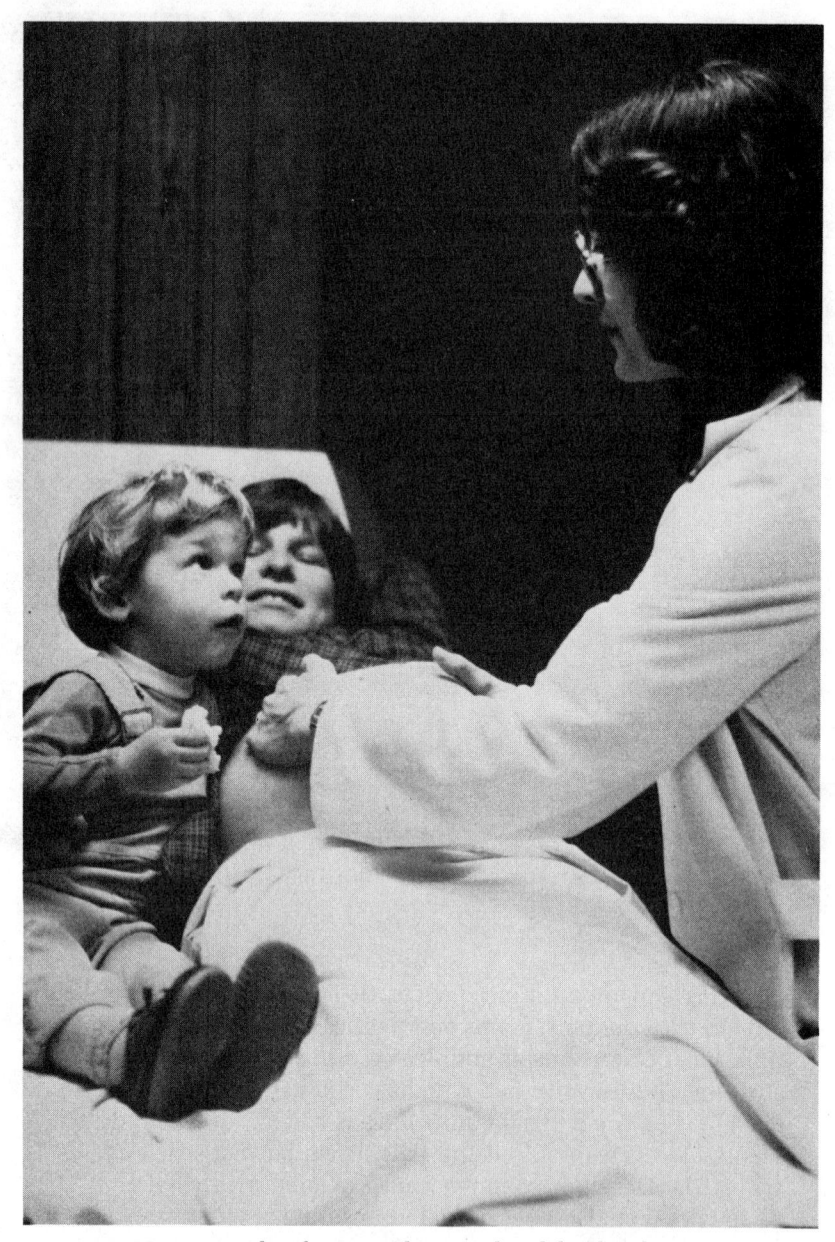

Nurse midwife completes a health checkup.

The state in which Janet works currently does not permit third party payment to nurses. The patients she cares for receive a bill from the physician group and the physicians pay Janet's salary. The cost of normal prenatal, delivery and postpartum care in the practice is the same whether performed by the midwife or by the physicians.

Pediatric Nurse Clinician

Linda Friedman is a master's prepared nurse currently in collaborative practice with about fifty physicians. Her practice is located in a large urban children's hospital.

Currently, Linda has a case load of 100 patients that she sees independently and an additional 100 Southeast Asian patients that she sees in collaboration with a physician. Linda performs routine pediatric checkups, often before school or before sum-

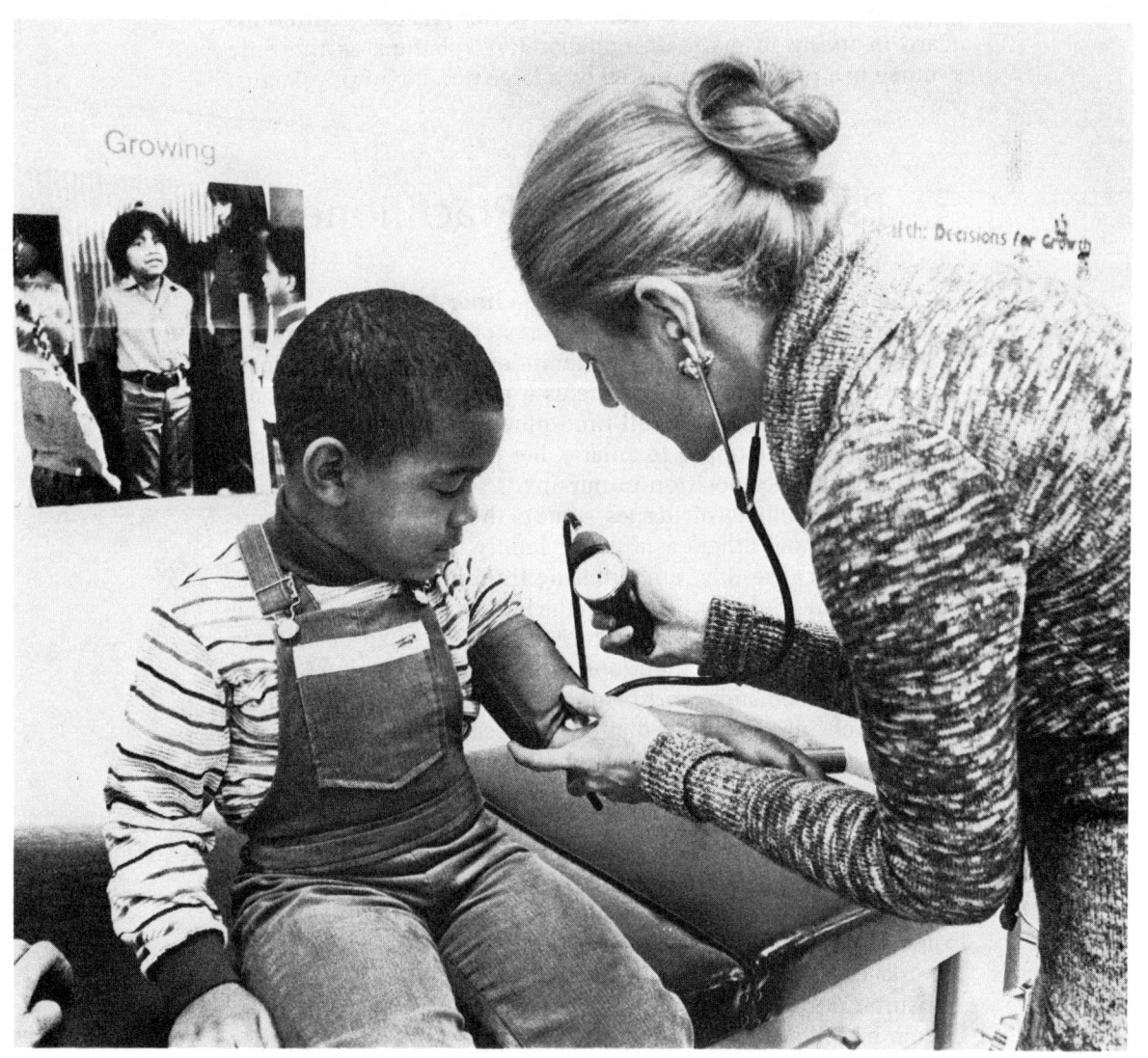

Performing a preschool checkup.

mer camp, and she teaches and counsels patients and their parents about obesity, and school and behavioral problems. Also she counsels couples who are having difficulty with their feelings about being parents. In addition, Linda also sees pregnant women before they deliver if she will be caring for their infants following birth. As a nurse practitioner she might also treat minor illnesses and prescribe drugs according to standing orders agreed upon with a physician.

Linda's satisfactions come from having children and their parents realize that their problems are not unique, that they are shared by many families. She also likes to see families begin to work on problems rather than blame others or feel guilty about difficulties their children have. Her greatest frustrations are in trying to maintain collaborative relations as the only nurse in a practice dominated by a large number of physicians.

Psychiatric Nurse Practitioner

Claire Towers, a master's prepared clinical specialist in psychiatric nursing, had almost ten years of experience as a psychiatric nurse before she began her independent practice. Claire now maintains a small practice as a psychiatric nurse practitioner while carrying a full-time nursing faculty position. In the future Claire hopes to enlarge her practice and maintain a part-time faculty position in nursing.

Claire sees clients of all ages, some of them individually, some as couples, and others as a whole family. Her clients seek her services because they are suffering from crises in their lives. Many are in grief over a death in the family, a traumatic divorce or facing difficulty in a job. Claire states that often her clients have a career crisis in their jobs. Sometimes this is due to a job change that demands more responsibility, or because the people feel stuck in a job they dislike, or because difficulties have arisen in getting along with others at work. Claire counsels her clients on how to cope with and deal more effectively with their situations and lives.

Claire began her independent practice by seeing people in their homes. She soon recognized the need to have her own office and now rents space, which she pays for according to the number of hours she requires. Since the state in which she works does not yet allow direct reimbursement to nurses through insurance plans, Claire is reimbursed for her services directly from her clients. She currently charges $30 for a one-hour session. If clients are in need of psychiatric drugs or hospitalization, Claire refers them to a physician who has his office nearby.

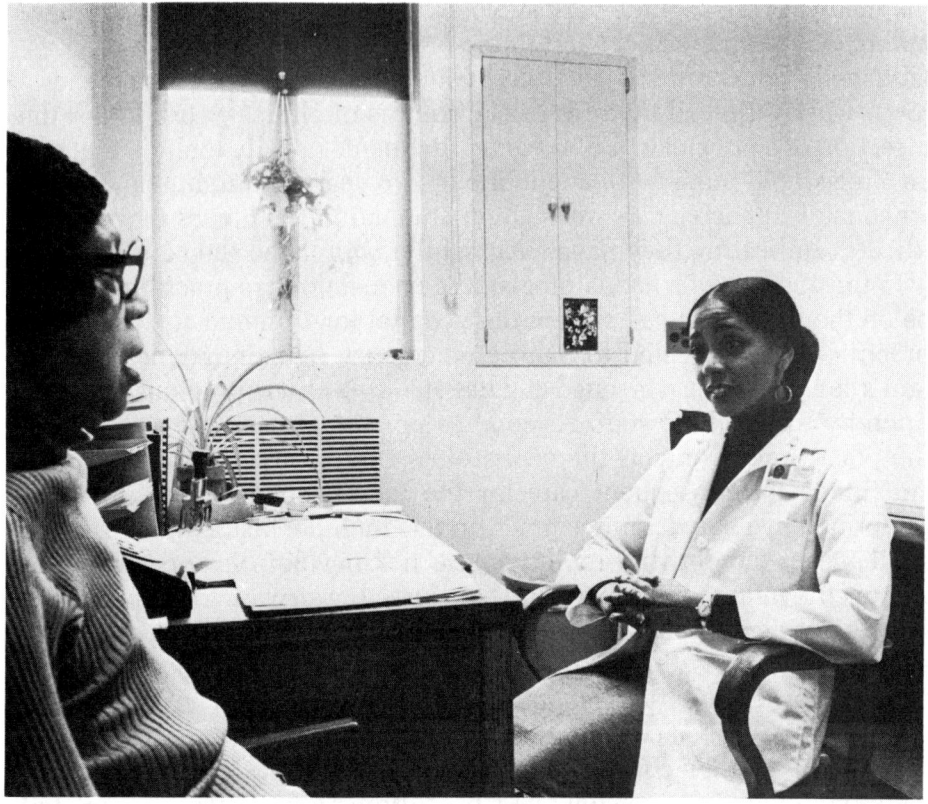

Helping a client work through her grief over her husband's death.

Claire too enjoys her practice. She likes seeing people change in positive ways that allow them to deal more effectively with the problems in their lives. She believes she plays a major role in her clients' abilities to bring about such changes. She also experiences frustration, not the least of which comes from the conflicts, resistances and anger clients feel when they must change their thinking or behavior in order to solve problems. This, says Claire, is the most difficult part of her practice.

Neonatal Nurse Practitioner

Neonatal nurse practitioners, like emergency room nurse practitioners, are not really in independent practice but are hired by hospitals for their expanded practice skills. As medical technological advances made it possible to save more very premature infants, the number of neonatal (newborn) intensive care units increased. The growth of these units surpassed the number of neonatologists (physicians) prepared to provide the medical care to these very sick newborns. In an effort to meet these manpower demands, neonatal nurse practitioner courses have been established. These courses generally include three to five months of classroom work followed by three to six months of clinical work under the direction of a physician. Entrance requirements usually include that one be a registered nurse with about one to two years of nursing practice in a neonatal intensive care unit. Upon graduation the nurses receive certificates indicating they have successfully completed the course.

In the absence of a neonatologist, the neonatal nurse practitioner may be on the unit or on call within the hospital for 24 hours at a time. The practitioner is expected to handle emergency situations when the infant's condition has worsened and use standing orders previously agreed upon by the medical staff. As soon as possible during the emergency, the practitioner contacts the neonatologist to discuss the interventions and plans for subsequent care for the infant. Some of the activities performed by neonatal nurse practitioners include: history taking, being available in the delivery room when a sick newborn is expected, ventilating the infant with a mask and bag, inserting airways to aid breathing and inserting catheters into the umbilical vessels. They are also responsible for providing thorough physical examinations, lumbar punctures and ordering certain laboratory, X ray or EKG tests. The practitioner is also available for consultation with staff nurses on the unit and to discuss the infant's condition with parents.

In some states the neonatal nurse practitioner's activities are regulated by state practice acts and so there are variations in their roles from state to state. In some cases, there have been difficulties regarding which department hires them (medicine or nursing), to whom they report and with which group they should identify and look to for support.

Certified Registered Nurse Anesthetist (CRNA)

Nurse anesthetists are another group of nurses functioning in an expanded role. Currently, certified registered nurse anesthetists give about 50 percent of all anesthesia administered in the United States. The nurses in this group have had up to two years of postgraduate education at one of 145 accredited schools of nurse anesthesia and have passed a qualifying examination for initial certification. Each nurse anesthetist must participate in continuing education and be recertified every two years.

The current requirements for admission to a nurse anesthesia school include graduation from an accredited program of nursing and current, valid registration as a professional nurse. Graduates of associate and diploma nursing programs also must hold at least 30 semester hours of college credit in addition to their nursing education, preferably in the bio-physical sciences, humanities and communications.

The American Association of Nurse Anesthetists (AANA) issued a position statement in the spring of 1982 calling for professional registered nurses to have a baccalaureate degree as the academic background necessary for admission to a nurse anesthesia educational program or school. The target date for implementing the baccalaureate requirement is 1986.*

Nurse anesthetists can administer intravenous, spinal and other types of anesthesia needed for births, surgery or dental procedures. Before surgery or a delivery the nurse anesthetist visits patients, evaluates their health status, and discusses and explains types of anesthesia that could be used for that particular individual during the surgery or delivery. During the procedure these nurses administer gases or injections needed to maintain the anesthesia. They are also responsible for carefully monitoring the patient's blood pressure, pulse and color in order to tell how the patient is withstanding the surgery and anesthesia. In addition to keeping the surgeons apprised of the patient's condition, they keep constant records of the patient's vital signs and condition during and following surgery, and records of the amount, type and length of anesthesia and other medications the patient has received. Because of their training in respiratory and cardiac functioning, nurse anesthetists are often called upon to resuscitate patients in intensive care, and newborns immediately after birth. Most nurse anesthetists are employed by hospitals, while some work for dental surgeons or in a group practice.

Nurse Practitioner in a College Health Service

A typical day for a nurse practitioner in a university health service encompasses both acute or emergency situations and routine health care. Students seek health care for physical examinations required by the college or athletic teams, allergy injections, gynecological examinations and contraceptive counseling. Emergencies include accidents, injuries and unexplained pain or bleeding.

---

*"Nurse Anesthetists Adopt Baccalaureate Entry Requirement." *The American Nurse* 14:23, 1982.

In general, patients are seen by appointment with emergencies being handled as they arise. When the student arrives for the appointment, the nurse completes an interview to establish the reason for the visit, then completes a physical examination and any laboratory tests that are required. The examination may range from a full physical examination to evaluation of a small area of the body. The nurse also has counseling and teaching sessions with students. During these sessions any prescriptions, treatment, teaching, such as breast self-examination, contraceptive counseling, nutritional counseling or other changes that should be made in their health practices are discussed. The average appointment takes from twenty to thirty minutes.

The use of nurse practitioners in university health services encompasses many components of the nursing role. The nurse has the opportunity to assess, diagnose, treat—under the physician's written orders—and evaluate the effects of the care.

The frustrations felt by nurses working in college health services are due to the lack of time for adequate health teaching and counseling needed by some students, and the lack of continuing contact with students regarding their health as they transfer or graduate. Satisfactions of the job include opportunities for promoting the health of a vigorous patient population. The role also provides opportunities for health teaching—through seminars and lectures—to the university population as a whole.

Career Advancement

Positions in independent or joint practice are not viewed as stepping stones to further career advancement in nursing, but rather as long range career investments. Some nurses do, however, maintain an independent or joint practice, have faculty appointments in schools of nursing and serve as consultants to local, state or national nursing groups; others also engage in research.

CHARACTERISTICS IMPORTANT FOR THESE POSITIONS INCLUDE:

- self-confidence
- leadership qualities
- ability to negotiate roles

- communication skills
- sensitivity
- ability to handle stress
- self-direction
- ability to function autonomously
- ability to make independent decisions

For Further Information

Write:

American College of Nurse Midwives
1522 K Street, N.W.
Suite 1120
Washington, DC 20005

American Nurses Association
2420 Pershing Road
Kansas City, MO 64108

National League for Nursing
10 Columbus Circle
New York, NY 10019

American Association of Nurse Anesthetists
16 Higgins Road
Park Ridge, IL 60068

Emergency Department Nurses Association
666 North Lake Shore Drive
Suite 1131
Chicago, IL 60611

National Association of Pediatric Nurse
Associates and Practitioners
Box 56
North Woodbury Road
Pitman, NJ 08071

Nurses Association of the American College
of Obstetricians and Gynecologists
600 Maryland Avenue, S.W.
Suite 200 East
Washington, DC 20024

Read:

Kendrick, V. "Nurse Practitioner in a VNA." *American Journal of Nursing* 81:1360. 1981.

Marchione, J. and Garland, T. "An Emerging Profession: The Case of the Nurse Practitioner." *Image* 12:37, 1980.

"Nurse Anesthetists Adopt Baccalaureate Entry Requirement." *The American Nurse* 14:23, 1982.

Nurse Practitioners: A Review of the Literature 1965–1979.
American Nurses Association
Publication No. NP-62

The Primary Health Care Nurse Practitioner.
American Nurses Association
Publication No. NP-61

Sheldon, R. and Dominiak, P. *The Expanding Role of the Nurse in Neonatal Intensive Care.* New York: Grune and Stratton, 1980.

Steel, J. "Putting a Joint Practice into Practice." *American Journal of Nursing* 81:964, 1981.

Thompson, L. "Job Satisfaction of Nurse Anesthetists." *Journal of the American Association of Nurse Anesthetists* 2:43, 1981.

4.

Community Health

While hospitals continue to employ nearly two-thirds of the work force of registered nurses, a study from the American Nurses Association reported that from 1972 through 1979 the greatest increase in the employment of nurses was in community settings. More nurses are needed to work in communities because patients are being discharged earlier from hospitals and because consumers of health care are demanding more emphasis on health services that prevent disease. The image of the nurse as an "angel of mercy," serving patients at the bedside is worldwide. Yet throughout history, a significant number of nurses have maintained the health of the public by working in the community, outside the hospital setting. They have been involved with preventing disease, prolonging life and promoting the well-being of people through organized community efforts. They have been influential in creating sanitary environments, controlling community infections and educating people in principles of personal hygiene. They have helped organize medical and nursing services for early diagnosis and treatment of disease, and aided in the development of social supports to ensure that every individual in the community has a standard of living that is adequate for maintaining health. The focus of the practice of these nurses was, and is, the health of families and the community.

At the beginning of the twentieth century, control of influenza, pneumonia, tuberculosis, epidemic diarrhea and other communicable diseases was the aim of nurses and physicians working in the community. Improved sanitation, nutrition, housing and the discovery of antibiotics resulted in a decline in communicable diseases as a cause of death and disability. These diseases have declined in the last 70 years, but other serious health problems have emerged. Chronic degenerative diseases, such as heart disease, cancer, stroke and mental illness, are now foremost concerns. The challenge for nurses and physicians in community health today is to develop a program which will be as effective in combating the diseases of the latter half of this century as were the techniques used against diseases during the first half of the century.

It is becoming increasingly clear that prevention or relief of chronic disease rests with the patient. Lifestyle and health behavior are far more important in influencing the disease process than any current medication. Many studies show the significance of cigarettes, poor diet, lack of exercise and alcohol in increasing the risk of acquiring heart, respiratory and liver diseases. In one study of 7,000 men and women, a research group found that men could add 11 years and women seven years to their lives if they followed simple health practices. The practices included eating regularly and not between meals, eating breakfast, getting eight hours of sleep a night, keeping a moderate weight, avoiding smoking cigarettes, drinking not more than one or two alcoholic beverages a day, and exercising regularly.

While chronic diseases and long-term health problems are major health concerns today, other social changes require a new look at how to deliver care to a community. An increasingly elderly population has created a demand for a different type of health service. Our mobility as citizens, with the accompanying loss of support from extended families, has increased the need for more humanistic and supportive health services to families. The high cost of health care has resulted in earlier hospital discharges, alternative methods of delivering services and consumers' demand for quality health care at a reasonable cost. An increase in sedentary high-stress occupations rather than physically taxing jobs, and rapid social change are expressed in a need for services to help people prevent, reduce or cope with stress. Yesterday's environmental hazards have shifted from control of microorganisms to the hazards of pollution of the air, water, food and land from human, industrial and agricultural activities.

Traditionally, community nurses worked within the established public health system. Today, they perform in a variety of places ranging from migrant workers' camps to the ambulatory clinics of major hospitals, through whatever agency or facility finances such services. Increasing numbers of nurses are practicing in health maintenance organizations (HMOs), neighborhood health centers, home care services and other areas in the community where health care programs have evolved. Regardless of the setting, the functions of nurses working in the community are much the same. The community nurse acts as a patient advocate, a collaborator with other members of the health team, and as a community organizer, consultant and coordinator of patient care.

As a patient advocate, nurses assist patients in obtaining what they require from the health care delivery system so that it is more responsive to client needs. The nurse may also function as a mediator among family

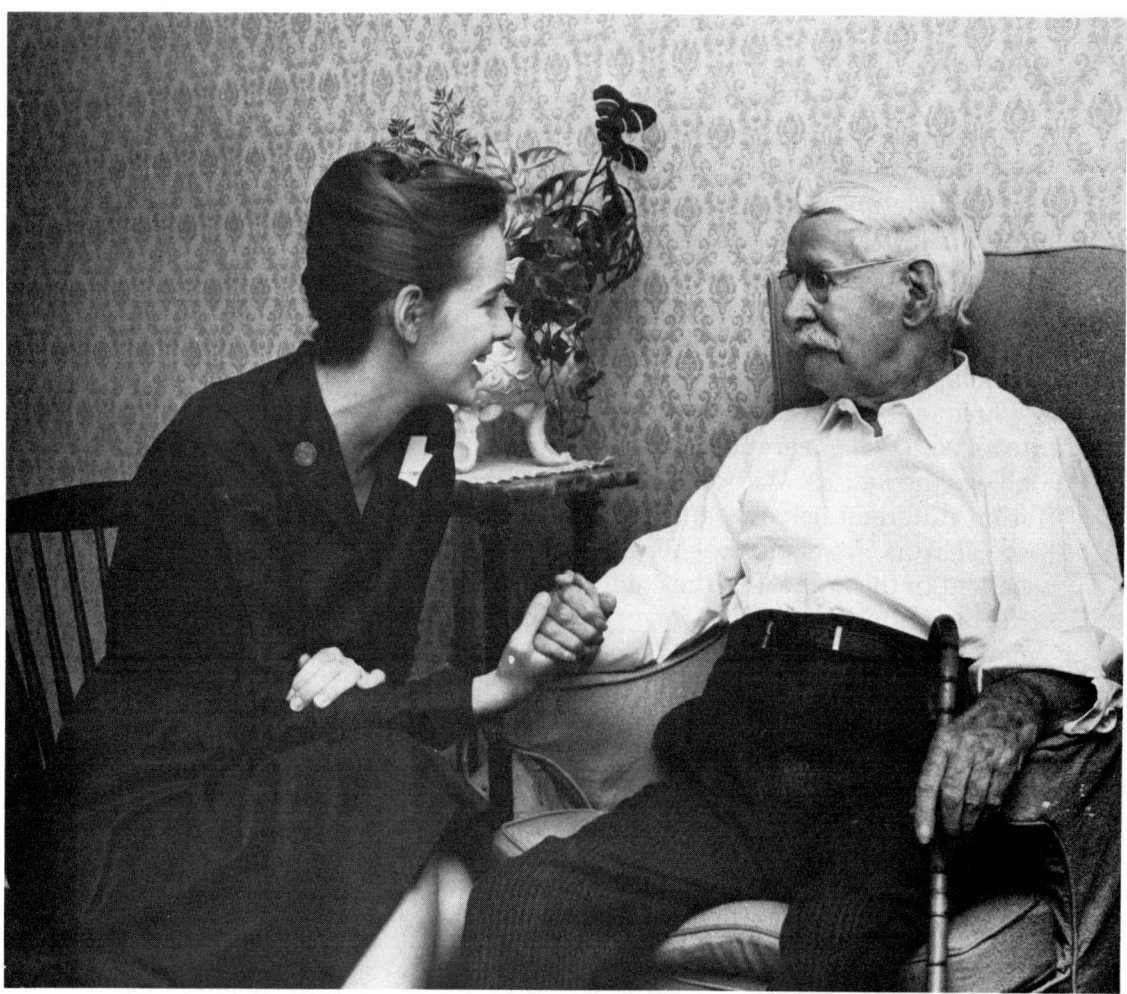

Encouraging independence in a senior citizen. (Photo courtesy of the Visiting Nurse Society of Philadelphia)

members or between the patient's interests and those of other community members. This is true, for example, in conflicts that disrupt group relations, such as those centering around differences in values between generations.

Within the health care system or within the employing agency, nurses work in collaboration with other nurses, physicians, social workers, psychologists, nutritionists, community aides, religious leaders and with the patients themselves. It often takes a lot of planning together on the part of all these people to help patients and their families.

Some community nurses use their skills to encourage community groups to develop their own health related organizations. These nurses try to help communities learn to speak for themselves and to express their own needs so they can make their voices heard in the agencies that determine how health care is delivered.

Community nurses often function as consultants to patients and to a variety of other people. Consultative exchanges occur with school teachers, legislators, probation officers or anyone else who has a helping relationship with the patient the nurse is providing services to. Many community nurses develop expertise in certain areas of care, such as contraception, genetic counseling, management of chronic illness, teaching strategies, crisis counseling, minority group ethnology and growth and development.

Frequently the community nurse is the member of the health care team who makes care accessible and who coordinates the services available to the patient. Without this, patients may receive duplicated service from different agencies and yet have some essential needs unmet. A social worker, school teacher and community worker may all see the patient in the home. But the community nurse may well be the one who fits their efforts together, sets up lines of communication and assists the patient in making decisions. These decisions might include things such as following through on a cancer screening test, getting necessary immunizations for the children and seeing a physician.

As an educator, the community nurse must be able to teach many kinds of people many different things. While the aim of teaching is to change behavior, such changes are not always immediately observable. The teaching performed by community nurses is of great value in preventing illness and is often the only preventive teaching that some patients receive. Sometimes changes in vital statistics in the community indicate the effects of the nurse's teaching.

As a researcher, the community nurse gathers a solid data base to improve current programs of care, develop new programs or apply new techniques in care delivery. Often the nurse is confronted with issues that are beyond or outside the scope of her own professional skill. Knowing the resources available to deal with a variety of problems and making referrals of patients to other services helps to resolve these.

As you can realize, to perform these many functions requires an individual who has communication skills and flexibility. It is a job for people who like to teach, solve problems and make decisions. Perhaps, above all, it is the challenge of understanding a variety of people—their values, culture and religions—that makes public health nursing an exciting pursuit.

School Nursing

School nurses have been an important part of the health care of children since the turn of the century when a famous nurse, Lillian Wald, started the practice in New York City. If you like to work with young people, you can join the 30,000 nurses who work in schools throughout the nation trying to improve the general well-being of the young.

Most adults remember the school nurse as someone who took heights and weights, checked their vision and bandaged minor injuries. In many places, all that has changed. Although school nurses may still patch up skinned knees, they also do health teaching, physical assessment, counseling and involve the family in health promotion. The reason for the rapid change in practice is the result of many factors. In 1972, federal laws gave pregnant girls and teenage mothers the right to stay in school. And in 1975, laws assured handicapped children the right to public education. Thus, two million more children were added to the public school system.

In one Philadelphia school, two nurses treat 150 youngsters with chronic conditions such as epilepsy, sickle cell anemia and retardation. In one three-day period, they gave 2,421 doses of vaccine to students. They also work with pediatric nurses in a nearby health facility to provide sex education and pregnancy counseling for pregnant girls.

Further, over time the health needs of children have changed. It is no longer important to be preoccupied principally with infectious disease. Today's emphasis is on a range of common ailments that may result in disability, and on more subtle matters such as behavioral and learning problems.

Usually nurses are assigned to one or more schools where they work on a regular basis during the hours when the schools are in session. The age and health requirements of the children vary, according to the grade range of the school, its location and whether it serves a handicapped or special group of children. In addition, because school health services are regulated by state and local laws, the functions of nurses may differ.

On a typical day, school nurses may meet with many different people to discuss the program of health services. It is important that teachers, principals and other school personnel be involved in planning and carrying out health activities on both a group and individual basis. School nurses must be well-organized, since they are responsible for planning their day so that there is time to carry out routine screening procedures, handle emergencies, make health assessments and see parents and children by appointment. In addition, the nurse may need to make home visits, or help establish special classes on health education both in the school and in cooperating agencies.

To become a school nurse, usually you will need a baccalaureate degree in nursing. Performing the role of school nurse practitioner, as described here, will require additional education through either a certification or master's program of study.

Many school nurses prefer to remain in their positions because they are satisfying in and of themselves. They receive yearly increments in salary as a result. Those who wish to advance to different positions usually assume jobs as supervisors or directors of nursing in their agencies. Some also take teaching positions to prepare future school nurses.

CHARACTERISTICS IMPORTANT FOR THIS TYPE OF WORK INCLUDE:

- an interest in children
- organizational ability
- communications skills

School Nursing for Emotionally Disturbed Children

It is a special person who works as a nurse in a school for emotionally disturbed children. This nurse must be able to react quickly in emergency situations, such as when children have reactions to medication or food, and to remain calm and in control when children are "acting out." The nurse, an integral member of the school staff, is involved with parents and community agencies and is depended upon for knowledge in many different situations.

This school nurse is often involved in the initial interview with the school principal and the parents before a child is admitted to the school. The nurse's role in this situation is to evaluate the child's medical regime, treatment plan and medication program, and to help evaluate whether the particular school has the facilities appropriate for the child's needs. Once a child has been admitted, the nurse is involved with teachers and the principal in evaluating the child's progress and in writing progress reports, which are updated every six months, on each child.

Much of the nurse's day is spent dispensing medications to the children and making sure that the medicine for each child is appropriate for his needs. The nurse is also in close contact with the parents to make sure the child's medication is being administered properly at home. The nurse remains in close communication with the physician as well, relating any significant behavioral changes of students.

Helping in the nurse's office is also used as a reward for appropriate behaviors in children's programs of behavioral modification. For example, if a student's classroom behavior has been acceptable, he may spend time assisting the nurse in administering first aid to a fellow student who has hurt himself. If the student has had a bad day and loses this reward, the nurse often spends time explaining to him why he lost this privilege.

The nurse acts as a calming agent with most of the acting out students and must have the expertise and knowledge required to handle these situations. Most often the nurse handles acting out students by just listening to them verbalize their anger. Many of the parents of these children are frustrated by their behavior. The nurse may decide to visit their homes with the social worker in order to provide them with support and to counsel them on how to handle these situations. Often the behavior modification program will be extended to the home and one of the student's rewards will be assisting the nurse in her office.

Since emergency situations involving drug reactions and seizures do occur, the nurse also maintains contact with the local rescue squad and local hospital emergency room staff.

CHARACTERISTICS IMPORTANT FOR THIS TYPE OF WORK INCLUDE:

- interest in working with emotionally disturbed children
- patience
- decision-making ability
- communication skills
- ability to handle emergencies

Camp Nursing

Camp nursing can be a fun-filled summertime diversion from a nurse's regular position, as well as an exciting opportunity for practicing in an independent nursing role. Today there are camps for both adults and children who are well. There are other camps that are specialized for the obese and those who are chronically ill with diabetes, hemophilia, epilepsy, handicaps and psychiatric disorders.

Before the camp season begins, the nurse (with or without the physician) may conduct a detailed first aid session for the staff during training week. In special camps for children with chronic illnesses such as diabetes or hemophilia, the instruction will include detailed infor-

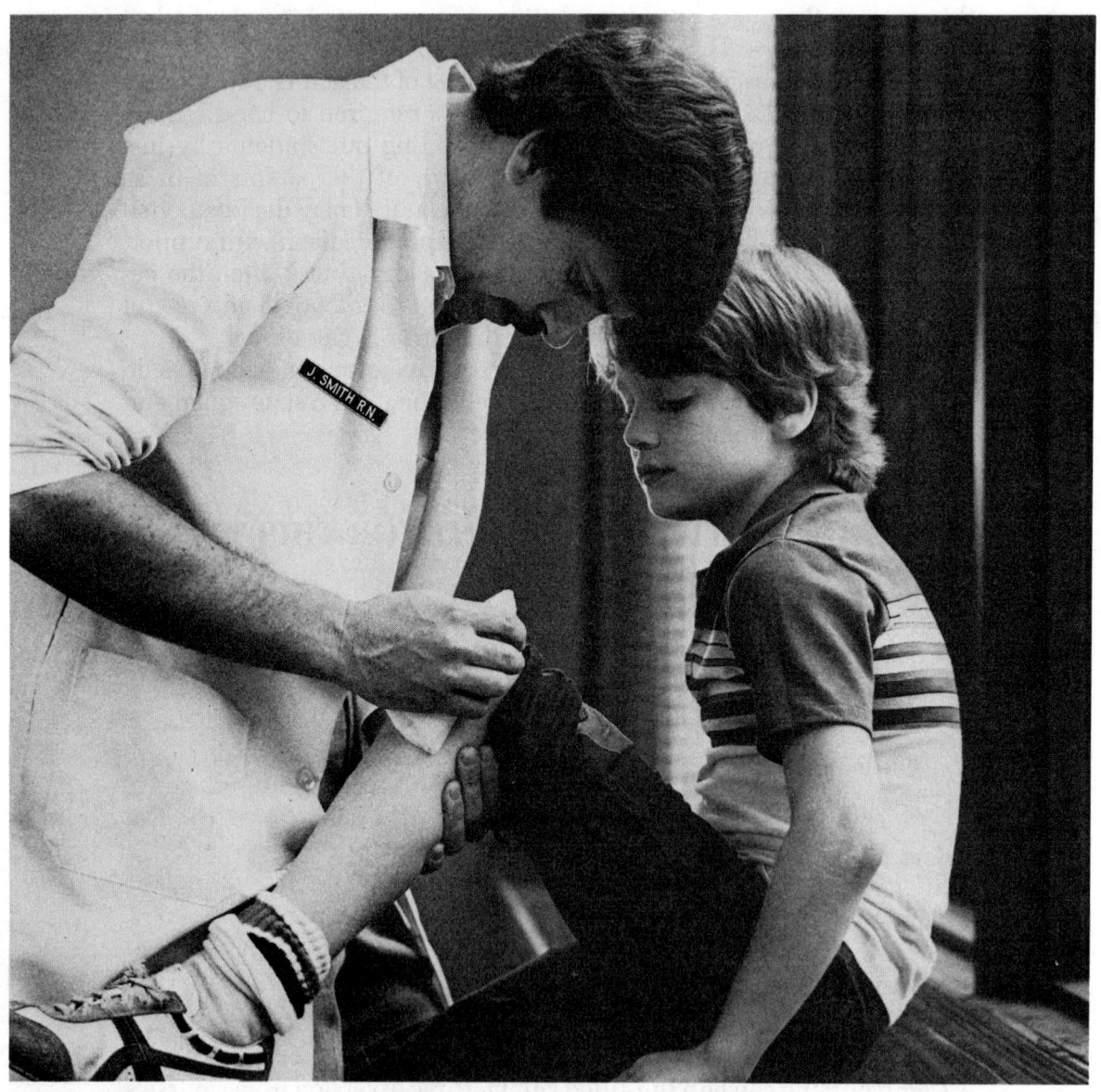

First aid from a camp nurse.

mation about the disease and its treatment. In addition, the nurse must assess the camp facility with respect to sanitation procedures, safety aspects and potential health hazards. Adequate first aid supplies must be obtained and distributed. For example, the athletic field should have a first aid kit that includes ace bandages, splints and cold compresses for sprains and strains.

When the camp session starts, the nurse usually performs physical examinations and compares the findings to the individual's health history. In some camps, physical examinations are more comprehensive than in others. Children's medications are collected and dispensed from the camp's health center during camp sessions. This approach provides the nurse with an additional opportunity to evaluate a child's response to medication as well as to continue health teaching. During the camp session other health programs, such as screening for scoliosis, may be implemented.

Throughout the camping period the nurse provides a number of services that are an inevitable part of an experience with outdoor environments and being away from home—emergency first aid for minor burns, sprains, eye injuries, lacerations, allergic reactions to insect bites and poison ivy, and, of course, homesickness. In some camps, nurses perform a number of other procedures as well. In one camp for hemophiliacs, the nurse performs venipunctures, determines the severity of a hemorrhage the child is having and gives intravenous medication following dosage guidelines arranged by the physician. In other types of camps, nurses make medical judgments in accordance with written orders issued by the camp's physician or medical committee. These orders usually permit nurses to dispense prescription medications for such conditions as external ear infections, local eye infections, allergic reactions and certain upper respiratory infections based upon the nurse's assessment of the person. The nurse takes campers to the physician or hospital for more serious illness and for emergencies requiring X-rays or laboratory studies.

Camp nurses develop and conduct health teaching programs. In camps for children with specific disorders, the teaching may focus on general health measures such as good hygiene and diet, as well as on treatment information, medications and maintaining an optimal level of health in spite of their disorders. For normal youngsters, the health teaching program covers first aid and hygiene related to backpacking, hiking and extended trail or sailing trips. Obviously it's a big help if you are an outdoor type yourself and have some real-life experience. First aid techniques and supplies to treat cuts, scratches, blisters, burns and sprains need to be explained as well as preventive measures to be taken for sunburn, heat exhaustion and heat stroke. The focus of much of the instruction is centered on having campers assume responsibility for their own health care—an orientation that hopefully they will carry home with them.

Camp nurses spend a lot of time providing hugs and reassurance to homesick campers. Frequent trips to the health center for vague reasons may be a signal of loneliness, boredom or inhibition in the new surroundings. Frequent discussions with other staff members help the nurse develop a thorough understanding of the child's behavior. A staff plan might divide responsibility for reassuring the child. The nurse might deal with feelings of homesickness, fears and dissatisfaction, and the camp counselor with building the child's ego by giving praise for accomplishing a task and by encouraging new skills.

At the finish of the camping session the nurse may perform physical examinations before the children go home. Any new or continuing health problems encountered during the session are recorded and sent home to the child's parents, and usually to the child's doctor as well.

While these are the general activities of a camp nurse, they will vary greatly depending upon the type of camp and the age and general health of the campers.

Camp nurses say some of the most satisfying aspects of the work are the pleasant outdoor surroundings and watching the campers mature and develop during the experience. However, they complain that they often do not have enough time to spend with individual campers, the pay is low and that they become physically exhausted because they are usually on duty 24 hours a day.

CHARACTERISTICS IMPORTANT FOR THIS TYPE OF WORK INCLUDE:

- love of the outdoors and camping activities
- independent decision-making
- ability to handle emergencies
- interest in health teaching

The requirements for the position include a license as a registered nurse in the state where the camp is located, an in-depth knowledge of first aid and an understanding of state health regulations for camps. Positions in camps for children with specific disorders may require further credentials and experience in caring for children with the particular illness. Salaries for camp nurses are generally low compared to other nursing positions.

Camp nursing is usually not viewed as a career advancement opportunity but rather as an experience in which nurses can have pleasant temporary employment and develop specific skills that may be helpful in other positions.

Rural Nursing

Rural nursing no longer means traveling by horseback to remote corners of a backwoods country, but many of its traditional aspects remain the same. It still means caring for the entire family and educating them in health practices so that they can better care for themselves. And it often means working almost on your own.

In rural areas people often live in isolation or great distances from their neighbors and friends. They may also live a Spartan existence marked by simplicity and frugality. Often they are strong individualists, very conservative and independent people who believe in the work ethic and frown on the welfare system. Most people are self employed—farmers, lumbermen, truckers, etc.—and have no health insurance programs. Often these workers are at the lower end of the wage scale and are not eligible for or would not accept welfare benefits.

In these remote areas, health care facilities are few and far between. The facilities that do exist are generally small with limited services. Hospitals often contain under 50 beds. Services such as mental health counseling and therapy and social services may not exist.

Nurses, working under standing orders or under the general supervision of a physician, are often much more on their own than their city counterparts. The nurse is often the one who sees the patient first in the hospital or clinic, and if emergency treatment is required the nurse begins it. In a rural setting nurses do a little bit of everything—emergency room, intensive care, pediatrics, maternity. Depending upon the setting,—farming, logging, mining,—they may see many patients with common types of accidents. Nurses in these settings also establish lasting relationships with patients and their families since they see the same patients and families through the years, socially as well as professionally. Nurses are usually very well accepted in these communities and are called on often for advice.

What rural nurses do depends upon the community and state in which they practice. In West Virginia and Kentucky, for example, an almost autonomous nursing role is possible. Other states such as New Jersey have very strict laws governing nursing practice outside the hospital. To find out the conditions you might expect to find in rural regions of your state, contact your state nurses association.

CHARACTERISTICS IMPORTANT FOR THIS TYPE OF WORK INCLUDE:

- ability to work independently
- decision-making skills
- communication skills

Occupational Health Nursing

Beginning in the first decades of this century, a progressively greater number of legislative efforts have been made to safeguard the health and safety of workers. The culmination of such efforts came with the passage of the Occupational Safety and Health Act (OSHA) in 1970, which declared that it was the intent of Congress, "To assure so far as possible to every working man and woman in the Nation safe and healthful working conditions, and to preserve our human resources." This law represents a landmark in the history of labor legislation since it legally recognizes three components essential to any occupational health and safety program.

These three components are the work environment, agents that can harm this environment and the worker. The legislation recognizes the worker as an invaluable national resource to be protected against endangerment from the workplace. Since its enactment, coalitions of labor, health and consumer groups have worked together to see that the legislation is enforced.

In efforts to improve the health of today's worker, the focus of occupational health and employee health services extends well beyond job safety. Many occupational health settings have evolved to manage a full range of health care needs in addition to medical emergencies. Many companies have developed health promotion programs. These vary from recreational pursuits and subsidized gymnasium or health club memberships to highly structured cardiovascular fitness programs. Some companies are associated with in-house health screening facilities and health education follow-up. Others have invested considerable time, money and resources in comprehensive health management efforts on behalf of their employers.

Kimberly-Clark is one example. They operate a health services center which includes multiphase screening, an exercise facility and an educational conference area. The multiphase screening available for employees includes a health history, physical examination, evaluation of height and weight, blood pressure, urinalysis, vision and hearing testing, chest X ray, evaluation of lung and heart functioning and blood studies for anemia, cholesterol and other blood lipids.

The company's exercise facility includes a 25-meter Olympic pool, a 100-meter track, exercise equipment, a gym area for calisthenics and other aerobic exercise, 1,000 lockers (500 each, male and female), showers, two saunas, a whirlpool and a lounge with vending machines. This facility is open from 5 A.M. to 9 P.M. Monday through Friday and from 8 A.M. to 5 P.M. on Saturdays.

The company's health education seminar topics include nutrition, weight reduction, breast self-examination, cardiopulmonary resuscitation and use of drugs, alcohol and other substances that may be addictive.

The health service center staff includes a physician, a master's prepared nurse clinician, two RNs, secretaries, receptionists, physical education specialists and technicians. Many other large companies have now developed similar programs staffed in much the same manner.

The objectives of these programs for management include reducing costs for medical care, decreased absenteeism and increased employee enthusiasm and productivity. Employees participate for many reasons which include exercising in general, recreation, camaraderie and health benefits. Some employees join in after being influenced by media reports about the detrimental effects of tobacco use, alcohol and drug misuse, excessive and unbalanced diets and lack of exercise.

Increased demands on occupational health services have paralleled enormous changes in the role of occupational health nurses.

In years past, the occupational health nurse functioned primarily as an assistant to the physician, helping with physical examinations, taking blood pressure, temperature, height and weight and treating minor emergencies on the job. Today most large companies with comprehensive health programs require that one or more of the nurses employed by them be prepared to function in a practitioner role.

Nurses working in this expanded role may perform preplacement and additional periodic physical examinations, see workers with minor illnesses and monitor the progress of employees with occupational injuries. They teach health maintenance, counsel workers with emotional, family or absentee problems and refer them to the family physician or appropriate community agency whenever necessary. In addition, they help employees with chronic illnesses to manage their illnesses in the work place. Occupational health nurses may also organize health surveys and develop or participate in health education programs.

In some companies such as Eastman Kodak, the nurse's role has also expanded in the dispensary. Here the nurse is responsible for making a nursing assessment and plan for workers who use the facility. The nurse's functions include interviewing, history taking, performing physical examinations as necessary and ordering laboratory, EKG and X ray studies. Following this workup the data (excluding X rays and EKGs) are used as the basis for a plan of care. Dispensary nurses may decide to treat minor diseases with medications consistent with standing physician orders or procedures, or they may refer the employee to the family's physician or to a community agency. All of these activities are carried out in collaboration with the dispensary physician as needed. The dispensary physician is responsible for X rays or EKGs to make a medical diagnosis and prescribe treatment. Nurses in the dispensary may also inform the safety department when they become aware of a serious injury or unsafe condition in the plant. Every opportunity available is used for health teaching and providing health guidance to employees.

Nurses working in these expanded roles have identified their satisfactions as seeing the same patients over a period of time, pleasant working conditions and helping workers assume responsibility for improving their own health. The frustrations they mention include workers with health problems who will not make efforts to improve their conditions and, occasionally, the routine of the work.

Occupational Health Nursing at Three Mile Island (TMI)*

While some might consider occupational health nursing to be routine, the person who holds the job of occupational health nurse at the Three Mile Island nuclear reactor, Peggy Hengeveld, finds it anything but dull.

> Peggy's actual title is Health Services Administrator. She holds a B.S.N. and has taken post graduate courses in health administration. Prior to assuming the position at TMI, Peggy worked as a head nurse in an intensive care unit and as a nurse on a cancer unit.
>
> Before Peggy was hired, there had been no separate health position at the facility. Health matters were dealt with by the Safety Administrator. Following her interview for a position under the Safety Administrator and her explanation of some of

---

*From Deborah S. Saline. "Occupational Health Nurse at TMI Radiates Enthusiasm for Health Role." *The Pennsylvania Nurse*, pp. 5–6, March, 1982. Reprinted with permission of the publisher.

Community Health 95

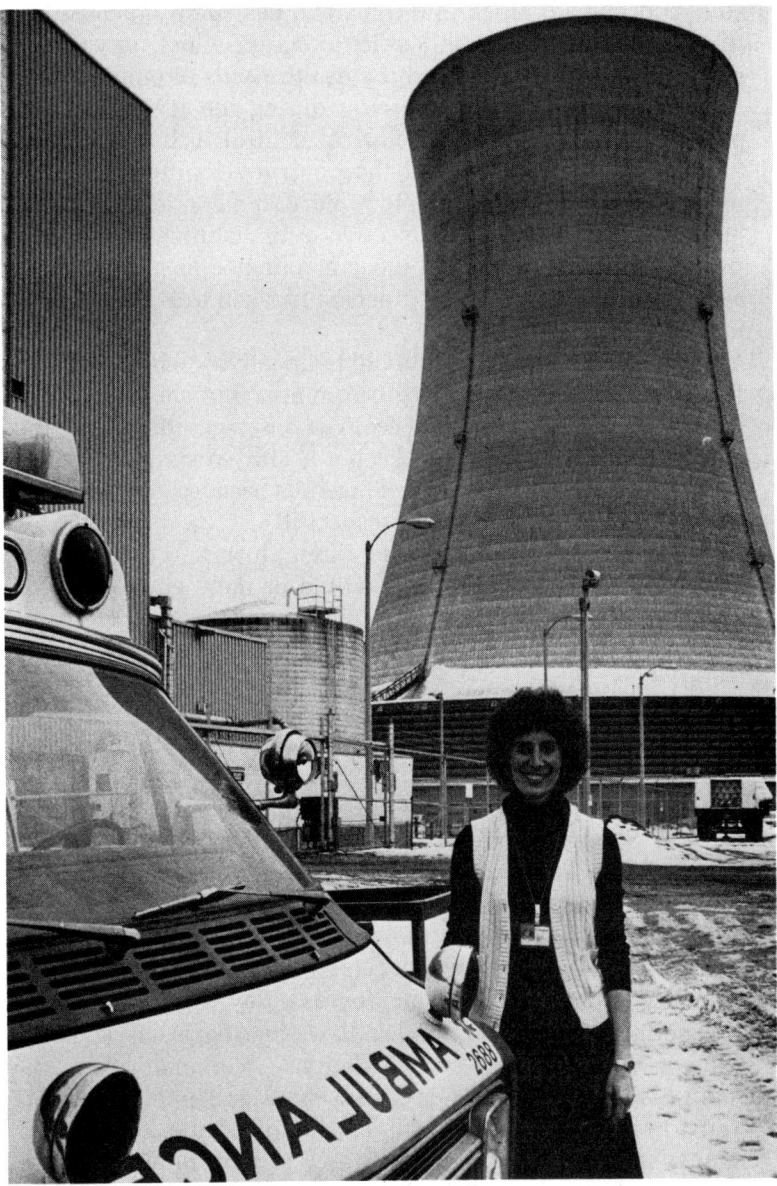

Occupational health nurse at Three Mile Island. (Photo courtesy of the Pennsylvania Nurses Association)

the services that a registered nurse could provide, she was offered her current position.

The Health Services Department at the facility consists of Peggy and a paramedic. Peggy supervises the paramedic, and together they are responsible for providing emergency medical care and equipment to personnel and for establishing procedures for the entire nuclear generating station. Peggy had been in her position for just seven months when the reactor accident at TMI occurred. Since that time, she has spent much of her time developing a health service program which is very responsive to emergencies and the health needs of employees.

One phase of the program is working the RADCON people. This is a group of radiological control technicians. One full day a week she works with the group developing procedures for dealing with a contaminated injury. If a contamination injury does occur, the first objective is to stabilize the injured person and bring him out of the contaminated area. First aid is administered and the injured person is taken to Hershey Medical Center.

Peggy does not fear exposure to radioactivity when responding to emergencies inside a restricted area. But she adds, "You must respect radiation and use T-D-S safeguards—limit the amounts of exposure (*time*), keep a healthy *distance*, and use proper *shielding*. Radiation is dangerous because you can't see, taste, smell or feel it—so you respect it!"

Peggy also teaches first aid to all employees, a requirement at all nuclear sites with one hundred or more employees. At TMI these employees include security people, operators, maintenance people, the RADCON group and the health physics technicians. She also teaches cardiopulmonary resuscitation (CPR). Since the accident occurred she has expanded her role to include employee health teaching. The Health Services Department runs a blood pressure clinic, a diabetes screening clinic and offers, for all employees who want it, a complete blood workup. She also provides counseling to employees about confidential health concerns such as problems with alcohol or personal problems that cause chronic absenteeism. According to management, since Peggy took her position, absenteeism has been drastically reduced. Peggy sees about 2,000 employees annually or about 15 to 20 employees a day.

In addition to teaching and handling emergencies, Peggy must know a variety of rules and regulations—workman's compensation, OSHA standards, insurance laws and nuclear regulations. Peggy says that her role "has allowed me to create an atmosphere in which nursing is able to help prevent certain types of illness through health teaching, or to diagnose them before they become life threatening." She sees her job as one of getting people back to work as soon as possible, keeping them from losing time and putting people who are restricted back on the job if they are ready to be there.

Peggy carries out this latter activity by serving as the liaison between the employees and the physician. Employees who have been placed on the restricted-from-work list come to her prior to returning to work. She evaluates their status, contacts the physician and discusses her findings. The doctor then decides on the worker's readiness to return to the job and Peggy documents what has occurred in the employee's file.

Peggy also helped establish the medical surveillance program that qualifies personnel for jobs at various plant sites. While abiding by the Nuclear Regulatory Commission's criteria for medical surveillance, the health team at TMI found the NRC criteria too basic and established their own guidelines for pulmonary, blood pressure, pulse, thyroid and eardrum screening. The criteria Peggy helped to develop are now being used at other nuclear sites. She is currently involved in stress testing plant guards as part of a trauma program being developed in which she will be able to administer drugs and intravenous fluids. Peggy's job is hardly dull!

CHARACTERISTICS IMPORTANT FOR THIS TYPE OF WORK INCLUDE:

- comfort with independent decision-making
- ability to communicate with a variety of people
- ability to function in emergency situations
- comfort with routines

The educational requirements for occupational nurses working in expanded roles are generally preparation at the master's level or a practitioner program in occupational health or family health. The latter must consist of up to five months of classroom work plus six or more months of preceptorship with a physician or nurse practitioner. Nurses in these positions may advance their careers by pursuing teaching or administrative roles in health services.

For Further Information

Write:

American Association of Occupational Health Nurses, Inc.
575 Lexington Avenue
New York, NY 10022

American Public Health Association
1015 15th Street, N.W.
Washington, DC 20025

Association for the Care of Children's Health
3615 Wisconsin Avenue, N.W.
Washington, DC 20016

National Association of School Nurses
7706 John Hancock Lane
Dayton, OH 45459

Read:

Archer, S. and Fleshman, R. *Community Health—Patterns and Practices.* Duxbury Press, North Scituate, MA 1979. (Chapter 1, "An Introduction to Community Health Nursing," by R. Fleshman and M. Jacobson, p. 3.)

Backman, H.; Packard, N.; and Reiner, A. "Camp Nursing: An Opportunity for Independent Practice in a Miniature Community." *The American Journal of Maternal Child Nursing* 1:88, 1976.

Bauer, R. "Family Nurse Practitioner in Health Services Center for Employees in Industry." *Occupational Health Nursing,* February 1978, p. 11.

Boutaugh, M. and Patterson, P. "Summer Camp for Hemophiliacs." *American Journal of Nursing* 77:1288, 1977.

Chaisson, G. "Correctional Health Care—Beyond the Barriers." *American Journal of Nursing* 81:737, 1981.

The Community Health Nurse Is Where You Need Her.
  National League for Nursing
  Publication No. 21-1601

Community Health Today and Tomorrow.
  National League for Nursing
  New York, NY, 1979.

DeMaio, M. "Role of the Primary Care Nurse in the Employee Health Service." *Occupational Health Nursing,* July 1979, p. 22.

Health Care at Home: An Essential Component of a National Health Policy.
American Nurses Association
Publication No. CH 9

Healy, B. "Exploring Ways to Expand Nursing Responsibilities." *Occupational Health and Safety,* November/December 1978, p. 44.

Kendrick, V. "Nurse Practitioner in a VNA." *American Journal of Nursing* 81:1360, 1981.

Little, L. "A Change Process for Prison Health Nursing." *American Journal of Nursing* 81:739, 1981.

Oda, D. "A Viewpoint on School Nursing." *American Journal of Nursing* 81:1677, 1981.

Ossofsky, E. "OHN's Assume a Prominent Role on the Health and Safety Team." *Occupational Health and Safety,* January/February 1978, p. 40.

Robinson, T. "School Nurse Practitioners on the Job." *American Journal of Nursing* 81:1674, 1981.

Saline, D. "Occupational Health Nurse at TMI Radiates Enthusiasm for Health Role." *The Pennsylvania Nurse* 37:5, 1982.

Standards for Nursing Services in Camp Settings
American Nurses Association
Publication No. MCH-8

Stephanik, B. "Nursing in Juvenile Corrections." *American Journal of Nursing* 81:743, 1981.

Stuart-Buchardt, S. "Rural Nursing." *American Journal of Nursing* 82:616, 1982.

5.

Extended Care Facilities

Does the idea of working with people over an extended period of time, helping them do as much for themselves as possible and at the same time maintain dignity in their lives, appeal to you? If so, a position in an extended care facility can give you that chance. Nursing homes, facilities for the chronically ill in rehabilitation centers, and hospices are all places that aim to provide this kind of care.

Nursing Homes

Patients in a nursing home may be there to recover from extensive surgery or trauma, but many are elderly and unable to care completely for themselves. Nursing homes are sometimes viewed negatively as warehouses for people, but innovative nurses are changing things and, as a result, the style of care is moving from custodial to rehabilitative.

One administrator of a nursing home believes that nursing homes require very special people because of the many difficulties encountered by the elderly. Nurses who work in these settings have the unique challenge of maintaining a pleasant, home-like environment for the residents while dealing with their immediate, long-term and terminal health problems. Nursing homes need people who can make independent judgments and carry out procedures without the help of the backup teams so commonly found in hospitals. This type of care requires people who can accurately evaluate a patient's condition since there are no interns and residents immediately available to consult. Nurses must be sensitive to the social, emotional and psychological needs of the residents as well as to their physical needs. They must be astute observers of physical changes because these can happen rapidly. Medications the elderly receive are often metabolized differently than they are for younger adults and can produce highly varied side effects. Additionally, the medications may mask other signs and symptoms of developing health problems.

Frequently nurses see elderly people who do not choose to be in the facility. Many would prefer to be in their own homes, or at least with family or friends. Men and women who come to nursing homes may be without family and friends, and confused, discouraged and cantankerous. They may have difficulty in feeding themselves, bathing and walking because of arthritis or poor eyesight. Chronic diseases may also have taken their toll. Yet, these people are at a time in their lives when recognition of personal dignity and worth are especially important. Nurses in these settings must know how to build on the strengths of their clients, how to help them cope with what remains of their lives and how to help them with a dignified death. Achieving this is one of the greatest challenges of modern nursing and is being demonstrated in the changes that are coming about through the practice and research of geriatric nurse specialists and practitioners.

Geriatric Nurse Practitioner

Geriatric nurse practitioners (GNP) are registered nurses who work in different ways from their traditional counterparts in the care of the elderly. Educational preparation for the role consists of three to four months of lectures at a school of nursing in addition to an eight to nine month preceptorship with a physician. These nurse practitioners become knowledgeable about the normal aging process and about illnesses in the elderly. While they work closely with the nursing staff and director of nursing, they often work more closely with physicians responsible for patient care in the nursing home.

Legal statutes differ from state to state as to what functions geriatric nurse practitioners may perform. But their special training prepares them to: conduct pre-admission assessments, perform physical examinations, order diagnostic tests, handle specific medical procedures, counsel patients and families, plan patient care and schedules, arrange discharge planning and conduct in-service training for other staff members. These skills enable the GNP to communicate accurate information to the physician and to discuss appropriate therapy. Geriatric nurse practitioners accompany physicians on rounds to discuss specific patient needs. According to a 1976 study, a well prepared GNP with good physician backup can care for 90 percent of patients' requirements in a nursing home.

Gerontological Nurse Specialist

A gerontological nurse specialist (GNS) or clinician is a nurse with a master's degree in nursing who has specialized in care of the elderly. The GNS functions as an expert practitioner, role model for other nurses, clinical teacher for patients and nursing staff, consultant and researcher. While the role of the GNS encompasses much of the practice role of the geriatric nurse practitioner, there is less emphasis on performing specific medical procedures and diagnostic tests and more emphasis on identifying common patient care problems, finding solutions to these problems and improving the total orientation and approach to caring for the elderly.

The GNS may give direct care to patients, working with those who present special problems. One GNS, for example, was confronted with an elderly woman whose constant scratching produced areas of bleeding and open sores on her arms and abdomen. Mittens placed over the elderly woman's hands only added to the problem. An interview with

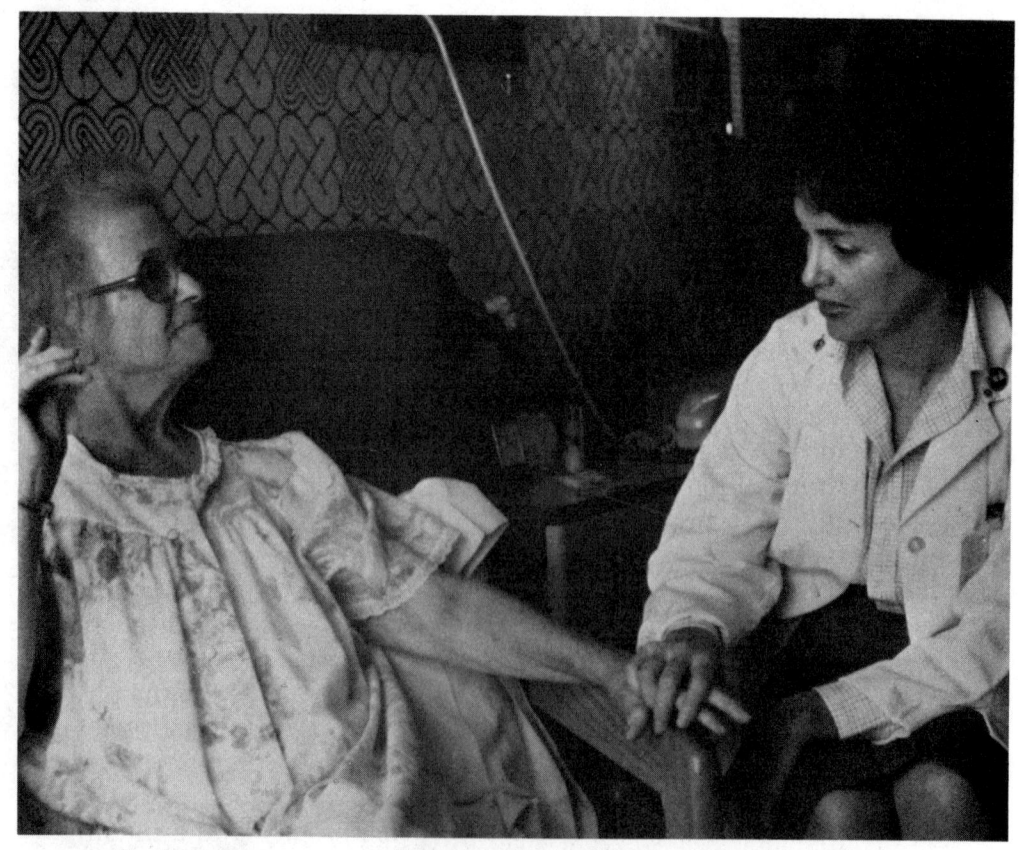

Geriatric nurse specialist providing direct care to the elderly.

the woman confirmed that she was agitated and confused. The GNS introduced a substitute activity for the woman by placing a necklace of brightly colored discs around her neck. The woman fingered the discs, her agitation decreased, and the scratching of her arms and abdomen was reduced. A small triumph perhaps, but one that is important to those who want to improve the quality of life for the institutionalized elderly.

Specialists may work with the families of the elderly, helping them work through feelings of guilt for having placed parents or loved ones in a nursing home. They may also help family members develop responses to patients who are hostile or confused or ask to be taken home.

The GNS also functions as an educator, developing programs and conferences for the other members of the nursing home staff. Topics might include the elderly's response to medications and their need for sensory and sexual communication. Stress is placed on topics which improve the care of the elderly, help them assume more responsibility for their own functioning and increase their self esteem and personal dignity.

The nurse specialist also acts as a resource person and consultant to the medical staff and the outside community. These nurses may initiate or participate in research related to improving care or treatments for the elderly.*

Nurses working in nursing homes identify some of the most satisfying experiences to include seeing improvements in patients' conditions that allow them to assume more of their own care and to feel greater self esteem. The slower pace of working in these surroundings has also been cited as a positive aspect of the work. Frustrations cited include problems in maintaining the hygiene of many elderly residents, and lower pay scales when compared to hospitals.

CHARACTERISTICS IMPORTANT FOR THIS TYPE OF WORK INCLUDE:

- interest in working with the elderly
- patience
- comfort with a slower work pace
- ability to listen
- communication skills

---

*Grey, P. "Gerontological Nurse Specialists: Luxury or Necessity?" *American Journal of Nursing* 82:83, 1982.

Rehabilitation Centers

In addition to nursing homes, nurses provide care to patients over an extended period in rehabilitation centers. The goal of care for these patients is to have them assume responsibility for themselves so they can return to the community and function as normally as possible. For some patients, the degree of functioning they can achieve is not enough for them to return to the community. These patients may require special treatment in facilities for the severely chronically disabled.

Rehabilitation is an approach to care that restores an individual to the highest level of function possible for that person. Emphasis is placed on the person's remaining abilities rather than disabilities. Because of the complex nature of the conditions involved, rehabilitation is provided by multidisciplinary teams. These teams include physicians, nurses and therapists—physical, occupational, speech and recreational. Psychologists, nutritionists, family and vocational counselors and chaplains may also be included. The center of everyone's concern is the patient, who is to assume responsibility for self-care or direct another person in performing care. The focus is not on caring *for* patients but rather on assisting patients to care *for themselves*.

This area of nursing may not seem as dramatic as some other areas but it is a challenging one, and requires a nurse who is a highly skilled and sophisticated professional. Many patients who are admitted to rehabilitation units are young accident victims who have just begun to enjoy independence or promising careers. Many others are older people who, because of a progressive disease process, have had several toes or a limb amputated. Still others are recovering from the acute phases of a stroke or other disabling disease. Each of these patients faces a period of adjustment and hard work in order to regain even partial independence. Adjustment to the reality of a permanent disability is often accompanied by feelings of frustration, anger, depression and guilt. This, in turn, produces a variety of behavioral patterns such as withdrawal, increased dependence, attempts to manipulate the staff, verbal abuse and lack of involvement in programs of rehabilitation. To manage these problems, health professionals need to be understanding, firm and mature. For the nurse and other members of the health team, long-term goals include having patients follow programs that will maintain their health and prevent complications, adapt to an altered body image and functioning, re-enter the community and resume social life, achieve an optimal level of independence in the activities of daily living, and resume employment whenever possible.

Rehabilitative problems are not always easy for the nurse to resolve. The most beneficial therapeutic program must be carefully coordinated to meet a specific set of priorities. This begins each morning as nurses or nursing assistants help patients prepare to begin their day. They help patients to bathe, dress and eat breakfast. These basic activities may be very time consuming, frustrating and discouraging for patients who have limited movement, coordination or ability to communicate. Routine nursing care often requires extensive modification. Brain damaged patients with severe memory loss or inability to speak require teaching adapted specifically for them. Trying to determine the emotional status or physical symptoms of such patients requires skilled observation and special communication techniques. An angry young paraplegic may lash out at the nurse who knows how to set limits on his anger and hostility over his predicament.

As patients progress through their day's schedule, periods of activity must be balanced with periods of rest. This may require frequent communication between the nurse and various therapists who might only see a patient during scheduled activity. In addition to coordinating patients' daily programs of therapy, one of the major responsibilities of nurses in rehabilitative settings is carrying out teaching with the patient and family in preparation for the patient's discharge. While discharge planning will involve the entire rehabilitative team, nurses function as coordinators and major teachers because of the amount of contact they have with patients and their families. Often the nurse will make one or more visits to patients' homes prior to discharge to evaluate the setting. In this way, required adjustments can be practiced while patients are still in the hospital. Following discharge, the nurse often maintains telephone contact with patients and their families during the transitional period of adjustment at home.

Nurses working in rehabilitation settings have identified the satisfying aspects of their work as seeing patients make the most of their remaining abilities and succeed in necessary readjustments to the outside world. Pleasant working conditions are also cited as a positive feature. Frustrations include slow progress or lack of progress for some patients and lack of family and community supports for patients.

CHARACTERISTICS IMPORTANT FOR THIS TYPE OF WORK INCLUDE:

- ability to work as part of a team
- patience
- interest in working with disabled individuals
- maturity

Requirements for registered nurses working in rehabilitation settings are sometimes set by the state in which the facility is located. Experience in nursing practice is preferred. Career advancement for staff nurses working in rehabilitation settings follows the same patterns as those of staff nurses in other settings.

Nursing Developmentally Disabled Children

The satisfactions, frustrations and tasks of a staff nurse working in a home for developmentally disabled children were described by one nurse working in such a setting. On a typical day her activities included administering medications and first aid, caring for sick children and teaching and monitoring health education.

> Early in the day she helps children bathe, dress and have breakfast. She also administers medications and teaches those children who are able to learn to take their own medications. The remainder of her day varies, depending upon the children's activities. Sometimes she accompanies them on field trips to stores, the zoo or parks, or sledding in the winter. Because of the children's disabilities, their involvement in the normal activities of childhood such as swimming, sports and cooking often result in injuries. So she spends much time administering first aid. She also spends a portion of her day taking children to appointments with the dentist or physician specialists or to hospital specialty clinics.
> Another part of the day is spent performing routine physical examinations on the children, checking for communicable diseases such as measles and mumps and coordinating their overall care. Since many of the children have multiple problems, physically as well as developmentally, they often receive services or support from a number of agencies and health care workers. The staff nurse's role includes coordinating the general care of the children to avoid duplication of or gaps in the services to a child from the various agencies. She is also in frequent communication with children's parents regarding care, treatment and progress. In addition to all of these activities the nurse instructs the child care workers on grooming, feeding and suctioning techniques, as well as on cardiopulmonary resuscitation. She also teaches classes in sex education to the children.

Additionally, the interdisciplinary team of nurses, physicians, social workers and child care workers write comprehensive plans of care for each child. The care plans are updated by the team every three months.

While these are normal activities, the staff nurse shared some of her lighter moments. She emphasized that these children are not sick but developmentally disabled, and prefer not to take medications. She usually has to "hunt" them down to administer medications. One hot summer day the children decided to cool off the nurse and threw her into the pool, medication tray and all. Another of her memorable activities involved a baby rabbit. The gardener accidentally ran over a nest of baby rabbits on the lawn, killing all but one. The children took the surviving bunny to the nurse to "make it better." She treated its wounds and fed it every two hours with an infant formula fortified with iron. The bunny lived and grew. The nurse and children let it loose when it was almost full grown.

Nurses working with the mentally retarded have identified one satisfying aspect of their work as discovering children misdiagnosed as mentally retarded to be, instead, emotionally or physically deprived. Watching these children progress toward normal life and knowing that they have played a significant part in the change is extremely satisfying.

Some of the most frustrating aspects of the work have been identified as dealing with members of the community or even the health care team who fail to see these children as individuals, each with their own potential, rather than as a hopeless retarded group.

Nurses working with the developmentally disabled advance their careers through further education and assume positions as head nurses and directors of health care in these agencies.

CHARACTERISTICS IMPORTANT FOR THIS TYPE OF WORK INCLUDE:

- patience and a willingness to wait for small improvements in the children's conditions
- willingness to be involved with children for long terms
- assertiveness in functioning as advocates for the children
- ability to accept the fact that children with degenerative diseases will die and will need help near death.

Hospice Care

A hospice offers palliative and supportive care so that the highest quality of life can be maintained for patients and their families when cure is no longer considered possible and death is probable in a short time. Insofar as it is possible, the goals of this type of care are to help dying patients remain free from physical and emotional pain, and functional until death. In addition, families are aided to meet the stresses associated with the patient's illness and death.

Hospice care is a team effort. A flexible, multidisciplinary team of doctors, nurses, social workers, clergy and often hospice volunteers provide the patient and the family with 24-hour, 7-day-a-week coverage. The majority of patients receiving hospice care are adults with cancer. An overriding concern is to control pain and frequently nausea that is a side effect of potent anti-cancer medications. In providing drugs for pain relief, efforts are made to keep patients alert so they can retain as much control over their situation as possible. Counseling and emotional support provided for hospice patients is aimed at an open expression of feelings about one's own death or the death of a loved one. Impending death is not denied but, instead, approached as the natural conclusion of living. Most hospice programs require that the patient and family be informed of the prognosis before the patient is accepted into the program. The reaction that the patient and his family have to impending death can then be approached as normal stages in the process of dying and mourning. As a result, expressions of guilt, abandonment and anger are more likely to be reduced, thus enabling the patient and family to concentrate on enjoying their last days together.

Most hospice programs aim to promote home care for as long as possible, although some patients may be admitted periodically to an inpatient hospice unit to give a respite to family members. If and when home care is no longer feasible, patients are admitted to a hospice inpatient unit where their usual lifestyle is retained as long as it can be. Inpatient hospice units may be located within a hospital or in a community facility. Inpatient units try to provide homelike furnishings, liberal visiting hours, family sleep-in arrangements and kitchen areas for individual meal preparation. Often patient's personal furnishings as well as other belongings are allowed in the setting.

Bereavement programs are also a part of hospice care. The trauma of the terminal illness ends for the patient at death, but it does not end for the family or loved ones. Bereavement and a sense of loss begin when the patient dies, if it has not already started with the anticipatory grief that is felt before death. Families who are helped with their feelings during mourning find that the quality of their lives improves greatly after the mourning has passed.

Nurses are a crucial part of the hospice team. They often provide the direct physical care and comfort needed by the dying patient and teach or assist other family members or friends to do so. They are frequently on call 24 hours a day and make visits to patients' homes in the middle of the night, if necessary. One nurse who is a member of a hospice team commented that often the members of a patient's family call when they encounter a problem. Usually the family has already done the right thing, but needs professional reassurance. Many times family members simply need reassurance that what they are doing is all that they can possibly do and that their contribution to the patient's care is valued. Family members call the nurse or have the nurse visit because they need to talk about how to deal with the patient's expressions of anger, guilt, depression or withdrawal.

Whatever the situation, the total family is the group in need of care. Much of the nurse's role is to assess whether there is support for individual family members in and outside the family circle. To whom can the members turn for help through the difficult period? In providing hospice care, it is the responsibility of the nurse and the rest of the hospice team involved to ensure that family members have a strong support system.

Nurses working in hospice care identify some of the satisfactions as helping patients find dignity and comfort in their final days and helping family members through periods of high stress. One frustration mentioned is not always having ready experience or answers to deal with dying children and adolescents. Another frustration is the occasional difficulty in reaching the other team members for consultation in aspects of patient care.

CHARACTERISTICS IMPORTANT FOR THIS TYPE OF WORK INCLUDE:

- interest in working with dying patients
- emotional stability
- ability to work with other team members and with family members
- maturity

There are no particular educational requirements beyond those of an RN for working as a nurse on a hospice team. Interest and ability to work with dying people is important. This type of nursing is not seen as a prerequisite for advancement in a particular type of nursing. Nurses in this role would pursue career advancement as would a nurse working in other staff nursing positions. Salary is approximately the same as that of a staff nurse. Availability of these positions is limited.

For Further Information

Write:

American Association of Neurosurgical Nurses
625 North Michigan Avenue
Suite 1519
Chicago, IL 60611

American Nurses Association
2420 Pershing Road
Kansas City, MO 64108

Association of Pediatric Oncology Nurses
Pacific Medical Center
P.O. Box 7999
San Francisco, CA 94120

Association of Rehabilitation Nurses
2506 Gross Point Road
Evanston, IL 60201

National Association of Orthopedic Nurses, Inc.
North Woodbury Road
Box 56
Pitman, NJ 08071

Oncology Nursing Society
701 Washington Road
Pittsburgh, PA 15228

Read:

Benson, E. and McDevitt, J. "Health Promotion by Nursing in Care of the Elderly." *Nursing and Health Care* 3:39, 1982.

A Challenge for Change: The Role of Gerontological Nursing.
American Nurses Association
Publication No. GE-9

Dobihal, S. "Hospice—Enabling a Patient to Die at Home." *American Journal of Nursing* 80:1448, August 1980.

Grey, P. "Gerontological Nurse Specialist: Luxury or Necessity?" *American Journal of Nursing* 82:83, 1982.

Johnson, J. (ed.) "Rehabilitation Nursing." *The Nursing Clinics of North America.* Philadelphia: W. B. Saunders Company, June 1980.

Leff, E. "Keeping a Promise." *American Journal of Nursing* 82:1136, 1982.

Minor, H. and Macauley, C. "The Nurse as Admissiosn Evaluation." *American Journal of Nursing* 81:118, 1982.

Nursing Practice in the Care of the Dying Client.
American Nurses Association
Publication No. NP-65

Perrollay, L. and Mollica, M. "Public Knowledge of Hospice Care." *Nursing Outlook* 29:46, January 1981.

Ringland, E. "I Am Proud to Work in a Nursing Home." *Geriatric Nursing,* September/October 1981, p. 359.

A Statement on the Scope of Gerontological Nursing Practice.
American Nurses Association
Publication No. GE-7

6.

Government Service

In addition to the wide variety of settings available to nurses in civilian life, the various branches of government offer additional opportunities for ambitious, talented, adventure-seeking nurses. Opportunities in government service are available in the U.S. Public Health Service, in various branches of the Armed Services, with Civil Service, in settings such as veteran's hospitals, as well as volunteer government programs such as the Peace Corps and Vista.

Public Health Service

The United States Public Health Service is the Federal agency whose mission is to promote and assure the highest level of health attainable for every individual and family in the nation and to develop cooperation in health projects with other nations. The agency is charged by law to do this. The Public Health Service's major functions are:

- to stimulate and assist states and communities to develop local health resources and to further development of education for the health professions
- to assist with improvement of the delivery of health services to all Americans
- to conduct and support research in the medical and related sciences and to disseminate scientific information
- to protect the nation's health against impure and unsafe foods, drugs, cosmetics and other potential hazards

- to provide national leadership for the prevention and control of communicable disease, and other public health functions

To accomplish this mission, there are six unique health agencies within the Public Health Service. They are the Alcohol, Drug Abuse, and Mental Health Administration; the Center for Disease Control; the Food and Drug Administration; the Health Resources Administration; the Health Services Administration; and the National Institutes of Health (see page 114). Much of the work of these agencies is carried out by a commissioned corp of public health officers. The corp is an all-officer uniformed service made up entirely of health professionals. They agree to serve wherever needed and are available to meet any health emergency in the nation or the world.

Pay, allowances and other benefits for the corp officers are comparable to those of officers of the Armed Forces. Benefits include medical care for officers and dependents, tax-free allowances for housing and subsistence, commissary, post exchange, officers' club privileges, and 30 days of annual leave with pay.

To be eligible for the corp, a nurse must:

- be a U.S. citizen
- have a bachelor's degree in nursing from an approved college or university
- be in good physical health

As a nurse in the corp, you might have assignments in medical and hospital services, research or public health practice.

Medical and hospital service assignments are available in numerous locations throughout the United States. The eight Public Health Service general hospitals and many outpatient clinics offer a variety of roles and experiences. The Indian Health Service has hospitals and clinics where nurses help the American Indian and Alaskan native populations in remote, underserved areas of the country. The hospitals and research centers of the National Institute of Health provide a range of new and challenging experiences in trying to improve patient care and treatment. Nurses could be assigned to the hospitals and clinics serving the Federal prison system or to the National Health Service Corps, which works in medically underserved communities.

Research assignments are available at some of the most respected and innovative Federal health institutions in the world. The eleven institutes making up the National Institutes of Health (NIH) study aspects of health and disease with the goal of easing, eradicating or preventing human suffering. This work is carried out by NIH research teams.

Nurses might also study, investigate and fight the causes and spread of disease throughout the world by working at the Center for Disease Control (CDC). Working with the Food and Drug Administration (FDA), nurses contribute to the safety and quality of the foods, medications and other products used by the American consumer. Public health assignments for nurses reflect a spectrum of responsibilities that range from teaching and counseling roles to health care management and administration. A nurse might be involved in developing new programs to make people more capable of managing their health, or working to improve health care delivery in a backwoods community. Student nurses may work as externs in the Commissioned Officer Student Training Program (COSTP) during summer vacations or breaks of between 31 to 120 days from school, and may gain experience in many of the areas already described.

Health Agencies of the U.S. Public Health Service

Agency	Function
Alcohol, Drug Abuse and Mental Health Administration	To reduce and eliminate where possible health problems caused by abuse of alcohol and drugs and to generally improve mental health of U.S. Supports research and the training of professionals in this area, among other functions.
Center for Disease Control	To provide leadership and direction in the prevention and control of diseases and preventable conditions (communicable diseases, urban rat control, occupational safety and health standards, among others.)
Food and Drug Administration	To protect the health of the nation against impure and unsafe foods, drugs, cosmetics and other potential hazards.

Health Resources Administration	To maintain or strengthen the distribution supply, quality and cost effectiveness of health resources to improve the health care system. Coordinates, evaluates and supports development of health professions and health facilities.
Health Services Administration	To provide professional leadership in the delivery of health services. Manages health care programs such as Maternal and Child Health, Family Planning, Community Health Centers, Migrant Health, Indian Health, National Health Service Corp, among other functions.
National Institutes of Health	To improve the health of the American people—conducts research and research training into causes, prevention and cure of diseases.

Indian Health Service

If the idea of visiting a family in a hogan or perhaps an igloo to provide health care appeals to you, nursing in the Indian Health Service could be for you. In these settings, you will need sensitivity and creativity to interweave tribal and traditional medical customs with new methods of health care.

This is just one of the challenging employment opportunities for nurses with the Public Health Service. Nurses may also work with the Indian

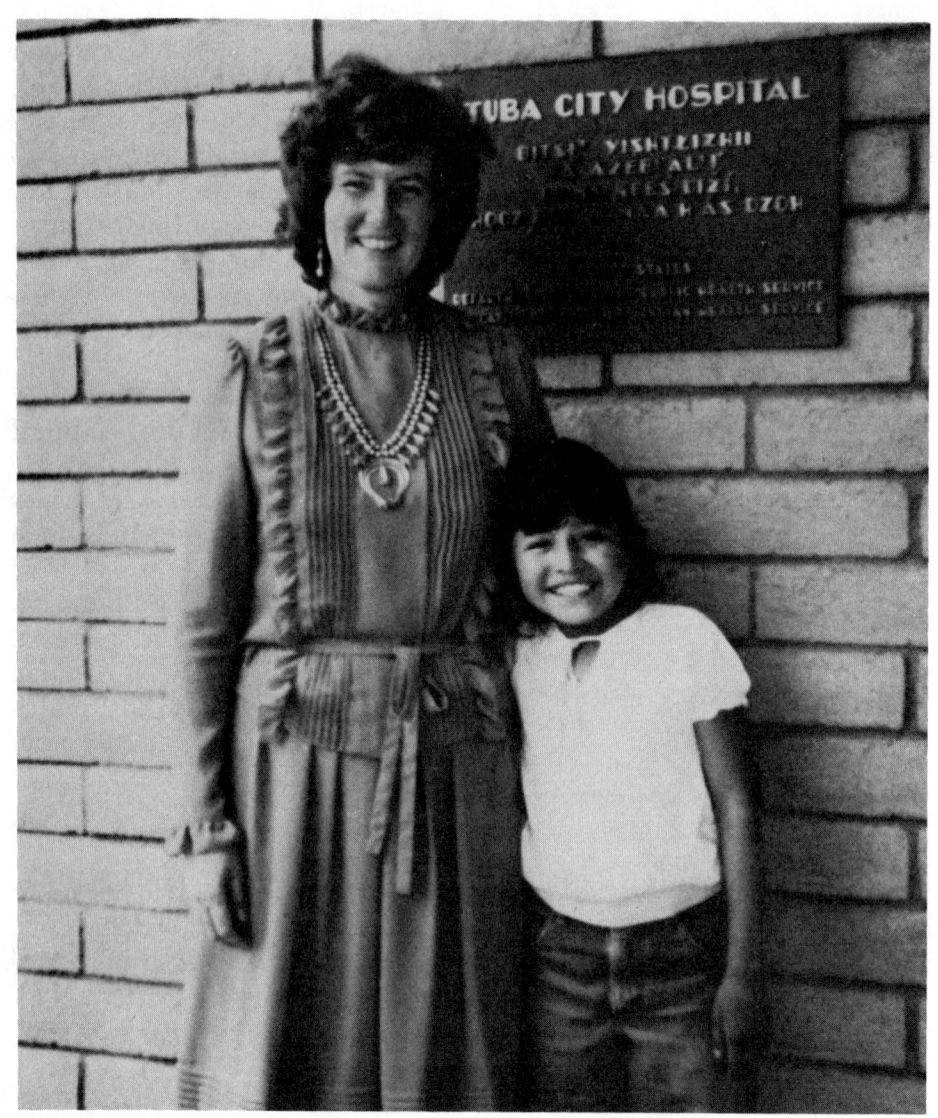

Nurse and young Indian friend.

Health Service through the system of civil service. Helping to meet the health needs of American Indians is especially challenging. Their health facilities are generally understaffed, and their waste disposal and water supply systems inadequate. This contributes further to the dangers of disabling disease normally present. The incidence of many diseases is greater in the Indian population than in the U.S. population as a whole. The incidence of accidents, alcoholism, mental health problems and suicide is very large. Infant and maternal mortality is higher than that of the U.S. population in general. Other diseases such as respiratory disease, ear infections, gall bladder infections and venereal disease are also higher in the Indian population. Life expectancy for the Native

Americans averages 65 years compared to the U.S. average of almost 71 years.

To meet the health challenges facing Native Americans, the Indian Health Service (IHS) operates 51 hospitals (ranging in size from 6 beds to 183 beds), 99 health centers, including school health centers, and 108 health stations. These facilities are located in 24 states including Alaska. The entire structure of the IHS is built to act as the Indian's advocate, while offering every assistance to the Indian's efforts in staffing and managing their own health programs.

Indian Health Service nurses have significant flexibility and freedom in their choice of work because of the variety of programs offered by the IHS. In the larger hospitals nurses can work in specialized areas such as intensive care, pediatrics, obstetrics, psychiatry and detoxification units. In the ambulatory care facilities and in the hospital outpatient units, nurses can work in prevention, diagnosis and therapy services for the mentally ill, alcoholics, diabetics, and those with tuberculosis, and ear infections, and those requesting family planning services. Opportunities for the community health nurse include providing services in the Indian's home, the clinic, the Bureau of Indian Affairs school and/or public school. Serving on tribal health committees and participating in community groups plays an important role in imparting health education as well.

Nurses in the IHS may also choose to serve in an expanded role as a family nurse practitioner, pediatric nurse practitioner, nurse midwife or nurse anesthetist. Experiences are available for nurses in research, as mental health nurse consultants, inpatient psychiatric nurses and nurse educators who provide training to allied health workers, such as community health representatives.

Further education and career development are planned for nurses in the IHS. Professional inservice training and education are provided for all nursing personnel. Postgraduate education is available. A one year's leave for education on full-pay status is possible after three years of civil service employment. The IHS provides a limited number of community health nurse internships. Attendance at professional meetings is encouraged and supported.

One nurse describing her experience working with the Navaho stressed the need for flexibility and sensitivity.

> Her days often began by visiting Navaho patients in their hogans. She arrived at the hogans in a van driven by a Navaho who served as a translator. During the course of the day she saw six or more patients. Her work included followup examination of mothers who had recently given birth, physical examinations of newborns, seeing patients with chronic diseases such as arthritis and diabetes and followup of patients who had traumatic injuries. She made a point of saying that Indians were treated in their homes unless they were very sick. The very sick

were treated in one of the local Indian hospitals or, if they required treatment not available locally, flown to medical centers. The Indians she worked with preferred to die in the hospital rather than in their hogans. Often in making her rounds to see patients, she would find a family had moved on to better grazing grounds for their sheep. A trip to the local trading post usually proved successful in finding the family's new location.

Several afternoons a week the nurse saw patients at satellite clinics throughout the area. At some clinics the nurse was the only health professional. Often in the middle of a large room where Indian women attended to their weaving, she performed physical examinations, treated wounds and ear infections, did health teaching and referred patients to the hospital. Many of her patients suffered from gall bladder problems due to their high fat diets, which consisted of large quantities of mutton and fried bread. Other health problems she commonly encountered were high rates of tuberculosis, accidents of all kinds, alcoholism and attempted suicides. At the end of the day she returned with her Indian driver to the local health facility. She enjoyed her work and encouraged others to try this exciting and challenging area of nursing.

Locations for Nursing Positions in the Indian Health Service

Indian Health Service Office	Area Served	Tribes	Health Facilities
Aberdeen area, South Dakota	Iowa, South Dakota, North Dakota, Nebraska	Sioux, Chippewa, Omaha, Winnebago	9 small hospitals 4 health centers 2 school health centers
Albuquerque area, New Mexico	New Mexico, Colorado	Apache, Ute, Pueblo	4 hospitals 4 health centers 2 school health centers
Alaska area, Alaska	Alaska	Eskimos, Aleuts and Thlinget, Haida, Athabascan and Tsimpshian	9 hospitals 7 health centers 1 school health center

Indian Health Service Office	Area Served	Tribes	Health Facilities
Billings area, Montana	Montana, Wyoming	Crow, Northern Cheyenne, Assiniboine, Gros Ventre, Chippewa, Cree, Sioux, Flathead, Blackfeet, Arapahoe, Shoshone	3 hospitals 7 health centers 1 school health center
Oklahoma City area, Oklahoma	Oklahoma, Kansas, Mississippi, North Carolina, South Carolina, Florida	Iowa, Kickapoo, Sac and Fox, Cherokee, Choctaw, Cheyenne, Arapahoe, Chickasaw, Caddo, Comanche, Delaware, Kiowa, Wichita, Creek, Ponca, Osage, Quapaw, Shawnee	6 hospitals 14 health centers 5 school health centers
Phoenix area, Arizona	Arizona (except Navajo reservation), Nevada, Utah, California	Apache, Hopi, Havasupai, Cocopah Pima, Mohave, Chemehuevi, Quechan, Maricopa, Yavapai, Paiute, Hulapai, Washoe, Shoshone, Ute, Unitah	9 hospitals 7 health centers 3 school health centers

Indian Health Service Office	Area Served	Tribes	Health Facilities
Portland area, Oregon	Oregon, Washington, Idaho	Bannock, Shoshone, Nez Perce, Confederated Tribes of Warm Springs and Umatilla, Ozette, Quilleute, Colville, Chehalis, Yakima, Puyallup, Lummi, Nooksack	9 health centers 1 school health center
Navajo area, Arizona	Arizona, New Mexico, Utah	Navajo	6 hospitals 10 health centers 11 school health facilities 34 other IHS facilities
Bemidj: Indian Health Program Office, Minnesota	Minnesota, Wisconsin, Michigan	Menominee, Oneida Wisconsin, Winnebago, Chippewa, Sioux, Potowatomi, Stockbridge-Munsee	2 hospitals 1 health center 4 tribal community health development projects
Office of Research & Development Tucson, Arizona	Papago Reservation in Arizona	Papago	1 hospital 2 health centers
United Southeastern Tribes Nashville, Tennessee	Florida, Mississippi, North Carolina, New York	Seminole, Miccosukee, Choctaw, Cherokee, Seneca	2 hospitals 4 health centers 3 health stations staffed by nurse practitioners

Indian Health Service Office	Area Served	Tribes	Health Facilities
California Indian Health Sacramento, California (Administrative)			

Career Advancement

Nurses in the IHS often advance to supervisory, teaching or administrative positions within the service or enter hospital or health service administration. Nurses may also relocate to other IHS facilities to advance their careers, if they offer greater opportunities.

Nursing in the Armed Services

As members of the Army, Navy or Air Force Nurse Corps, nurses have ranks as officers. They have chances to advance their careers through new clinical experiences and through changing nursing specialities or geographical locations, without losing seniority. The Armed Services offers opportunities for continued education and travel. In addition, nurses receive excellent personal benefits, including 30 days paid vacation each year, free medical and dental care, retirement benefits, moving and travel costs and uniform allowances.

Qualifications

Qualifications for a commission in the nurse corp vary from one branch of the armed services to another. To become an Army nurse, a minimum of a Bachelor of Science in Nursing from an accredited college or university is necessary. The Navy Nurse Corp requires a bachelor's degree from an accredited nursing program of at least 108 academic weeks' duration (excluding vacation periods), plus a minimum of one year's nursing experience. The Air Force requires graduation from an accredited school of nursing acceptable to the Surgeon General of the United States Air Force. All branches of the service require nurses to carry a current registration in one state, the District of Columbia or a territory of the United States. They also require that nurses be in good physical health. The minimum age requirement for the Air Force is 18 years, for the Navy, 20, and for the Army, 21.

Orientation

All branches of the armed services provide a course of orientation. Army nurses attend a five-week Officer Basic Orientation Course at Fort Sam Houston, San Antonio, Texas. Here nurses attend lectures, conferences, films and demonstrations which cover everything from military customs to management of mass casualties. They also spend a few days in a simulated combat area in preparation for using their skills under combat conditions.

Navy nurses attend a five and one-half week Officer Indoctrination Program in Newport, Rhode Island. Here they learn Navy customs, protocol, procedures and the duties and responsibilities of a naval officer. Program topics include military law, naval history, leadership, personnel policies, organization of the Navy Medical Department and physical education.

The Air Force officer's orientation program is two weeks long and held at Sheppard Air Force Base, Wichita Falls, Texas. The program includes information about the Air Force mission, structure and operation of the Medical Service, Air Force traditions and customs and the nurse's role as an Air Force officer.

Following the orientation program, armed services nurses usually begin their assignments in armed services hospitals in the United States.

Nursing Assignments

The Army Medical Department is one of the largest comprehensive systems of health care in the world. The system provides care for more than three million men and women active in the army, their families,

Government Service 123

and retired servicemen and women and their families. Over 5,000 army physicians and nurses practice in 48 hospitals in eight countries. Nurses who receive overseas assignments on a first or subsequent tour of duty may be stationed in Germany, Hawaii, Italy, Korea, Belgium or Alaska.

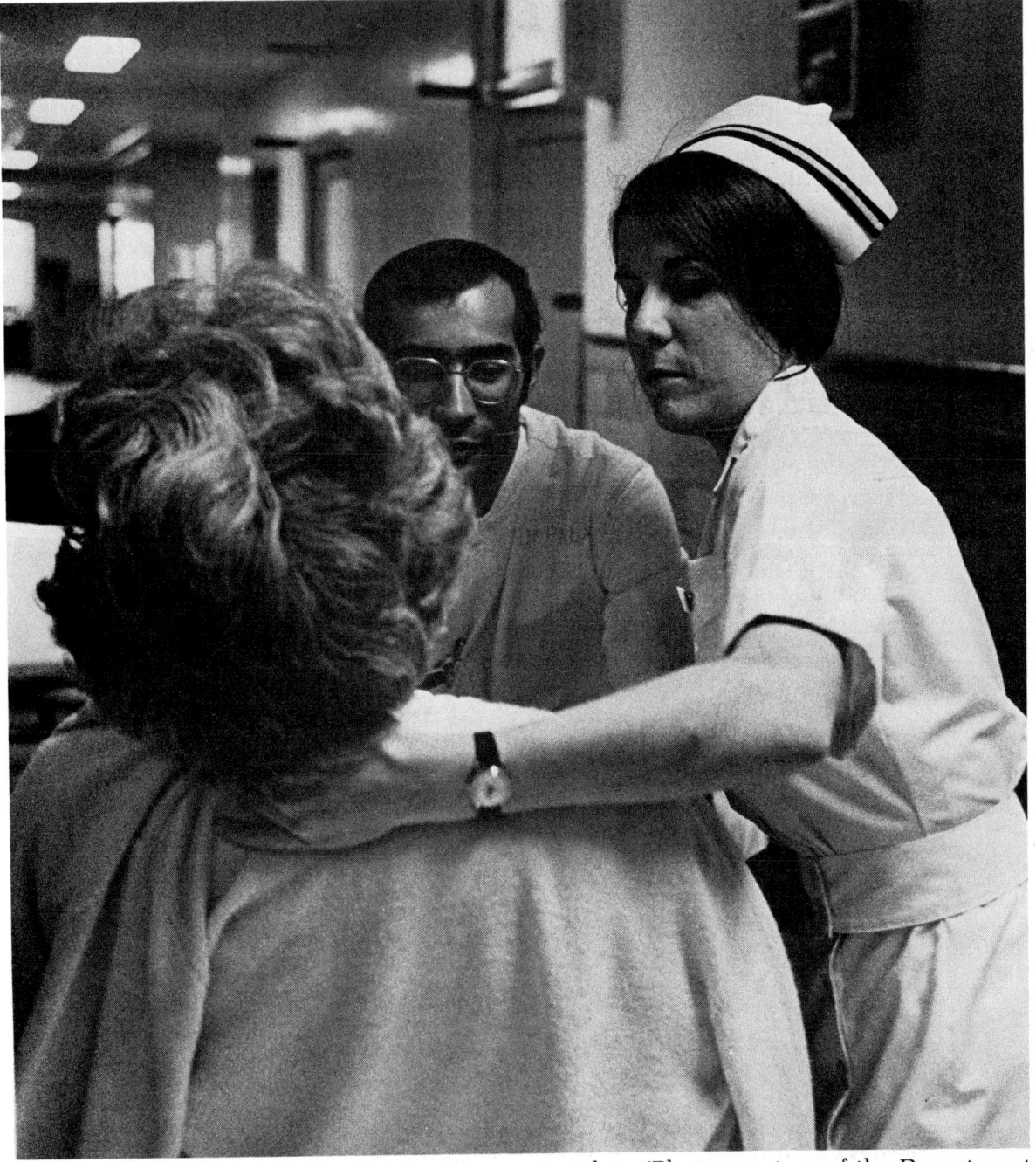

Navy nurse helping a patient lie down on a stretcher. (Photo courtesy of the Department of Defense)

In addition to serving in one of the army's hospitals, nurses may be sent anywhere in the world to aid victims of natural disasters. Army nurses, for example, were among the first to arrive on the scene and participate in relief operations for earthquake victims in Chile, Iran, Yugoslavia, Guatemala and Alaska.

Newly commissioned Navy nurses are assigned to selected naval hospitals within the United States. Following a period of orientation, which includes patient care management, interdepartmental relationships and procedural skills, the nurses assume charge of a ward. They are then responsible for the total care of patients, management and supervision of the ward, and supervision and instruction of the hospital corps personnel. Navy nurses are eligible for overseas assignments when they have completed one tour of duty stateside. Overseas stations for Navy

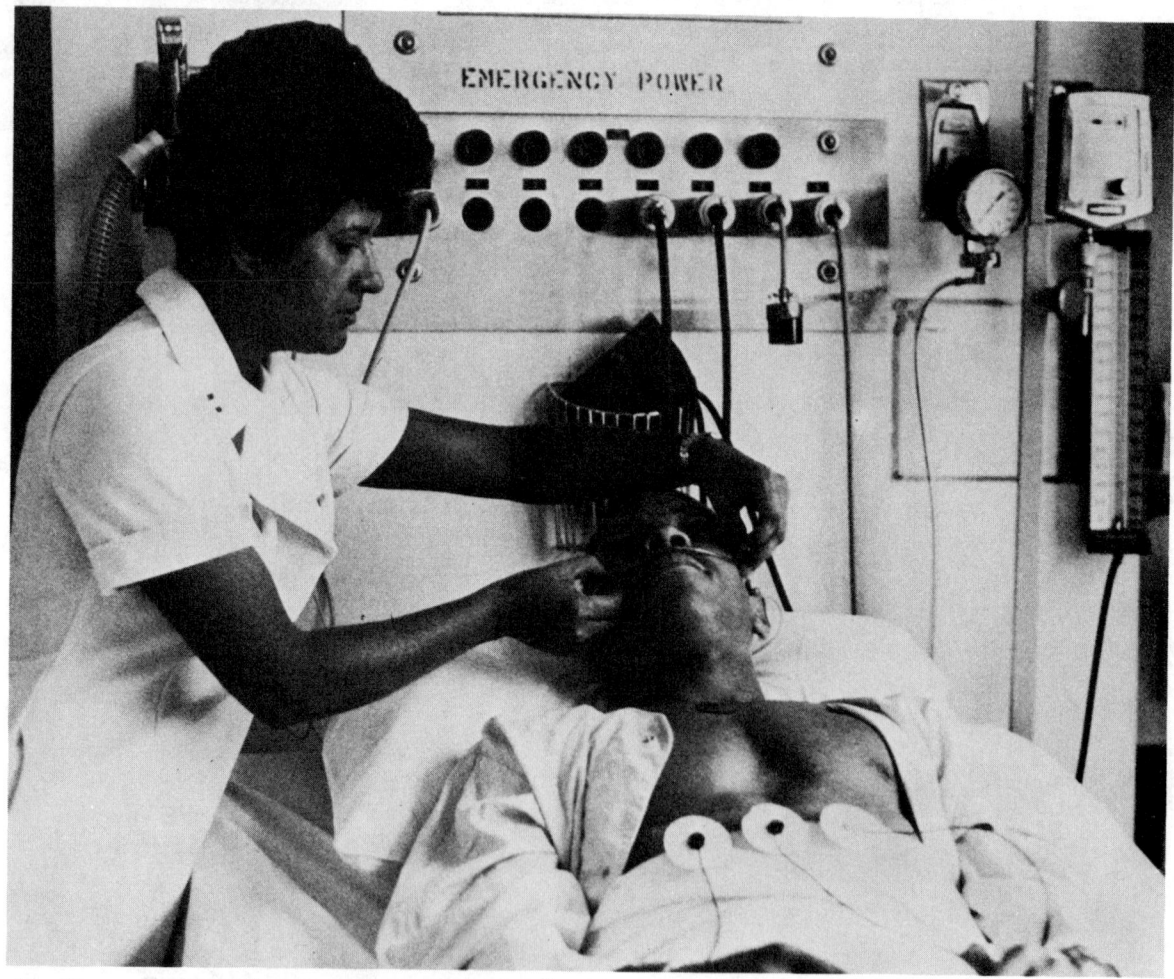

Air Force nurse adjusting the oxygen intake of a patient in an intensive care unit. (Photo courtesy of the Department of Defense)

nurses are located in Guam, Japan, Italy, Puerto Rico, the Philippines, Alaska, Taiwan, Sardinia, Western Australia, Egypt, Korea, Hawaii, Cuba, Spain, Iceland, Newfoundland, Bermuda and Midway Island in the Pacific.

Like most of their Army and Navy counterparts, Air Force nurses begin their assignments at a hospital within the United States. The size of the hospital may range from 25 to 1,000 beds. While there are more than 115 Air Force medical facilities worldwide, the Air Force health care system in the United States is divided into six geographical regions. Many newly commissioned nurses are assigned to one of these six Air Force medical centers. Each region is served by a large medical center, hospitals and clinics. All Air Force health facilities serve the communities within which they are based. The regional medical centers provide specialized care, consultation services and operational support for the smaller facilities in their area. If patients in overseas or other military hospitals need the specialized care provided in any one of these centers, they are flown to the nearest center that offers the required services.

In addition to their assignment to a hospital, nurses in the armed services, like their civilian counterparts, work in clinical specialty areas of nursing. Some of these are neurosurgery, psychiatry, obstetrics and gynecology, medicine and surgery, intensive care, pediatrics, operating rooms, orthopedics, renal dialysis, infection control, emergency room, cancer units, research and ambulatory care.

For nurses interested in practicing in an expanded role, armed services' practitioner programs are available in a number of areas of nursing. The Army offers nurse practitioner courses in pediatrics, adult medical-surgical health care, and obstetrics and gynecology. They also offer clinical specialty courses in intensive care, operating room nursing, community health and environmental science, psychiatric mental health nursing, anesthesiology and nurse midwifery.

The Navy sponsors nurses practitioner programs in obstetrics and gynecology, pediatrics, family practice, operating room technique and training of nurse anesthetists.

The Air Force offers courses in expanded nursing roles such as obstetric and gynecologic nurse practitioner, pediatric nurse practitioner, flight nurse, critical care nurse, nurse anesthetist, environmental health nurse, manager of nursing services and midwifery.

All branches of the armed services nurse corp encourage nurses to pursue further formal education and will pay partial tuition for part-time study while nurses are on full-time assignment. In addition, with a commitment to further service obligations some nurses receive full tuition and fees plus their service salaries while they study full-time for a higher degree in nursing. As students, nurses may participate in ROTC programs, in which all or part of a collegiate program in nursing is financed by the service.

Army School Nurse

A few civilian positions are also available in some armed forces bases overseas.

> One nurse whose husband was stationed in Germany shared her work as a nurse in an Army school. Her activities included health screening, vision and hearing testing, routine physical examinations, evaluation of immunizations and testing for tuberculosis. She cared for children with sudden illnesses, fevers, rashes and sudden vomiting, until the children could be seen by the physician. She also did health teaching, the activity she found most satisfying. She taught concepts of health and health care practices from the lower grades through high school. In high school she also taught sex education.
>
> Another satisfaction she felt working in this role was the opportunity to work and live in a foreign country, but at the same time work for the U.S. govenment with the accompanying protections and privileges.
>
> There were frustrations as well. Since Army children often relocate, they sometimes have difficulty establishing roots and relationships with others. She encountered many discipline and emotional problems in the children. There were also communication problems with some service children who had been born and raised in other countries and who were just learning English.

Civil Service

Nurses in civil service enjoy a variety of work experiences available in many geographical locations, and good salaries and employee benefits. Eligibility for employment through the civil service requires:

- U.S. citizenship
- graduation from an approved school of nursing
- current registration as a nurse in any state or territory of the U.S. or the District of Columbia
- satisfactory health

As noted previously, nurses may work in the Indian Health Services as a civil servant as well as under the United States Public Health Service. Many nurses in civil service also work as nurses within the Veterans Administration (VA).

Veterans Administration

The VA was established in 1930 to administer Federal programs which provide assistance to the nation's veterans. Today, the VA operates the nation's largest health care system, made up of over 170 medical centers located throughout the country. In addition, there are more than 230 outpatient clinics and other facilities, most operating in conjunction with medical centers. Health care facilities range in size from 100 beds to over 2,000 beds. About one million hospitalized patients are treated each year.

To provide veterans with the best medical care available, the VA has established extensive research and educational programs. Most VA medical centers are affiliated with medical and nursing schools and all are linked with at least one institution of higher learning for the training of medical and allied health personnel.

VA nurses are assuming an increasingly important role in planning, implementing and evaluating the care given to veterans. These nurses work in a variety of general and specialized patient treatment programs. In addition to medical, surgical and psychiatric units, VA nurses are employed in specialized services, including alcohol and drug dependence treatment units, clinics for the blind, centers for epileptics, hemodialysis and home dialysis units, intensive and coronary care units, organ transplant centers and spinal cord injury units. Nurses with advanced education work in expanded roles in prehospital and posthospital care, such as ambulatory care settings, nursing home care units, day treatment centers, outpatient clinics and hospital-based home care programs. Other nurses use their specialized skills and knowledge in the areas of research, education and administration. The VA has doctorally-prepared nurse researchers whose research at the health care facilities is aimed at improving the quality of patient care. Other nurses participate in continuing education programs with nursing groups in the local community, and help teach medical and nursing students who affiliate at the institution. Many of these nurses hold faculty appointments at the affiliating schools of nursing.

Programs of continuing education are available for VA nurses. Specialized courses prepare them for providing care in specialty units such

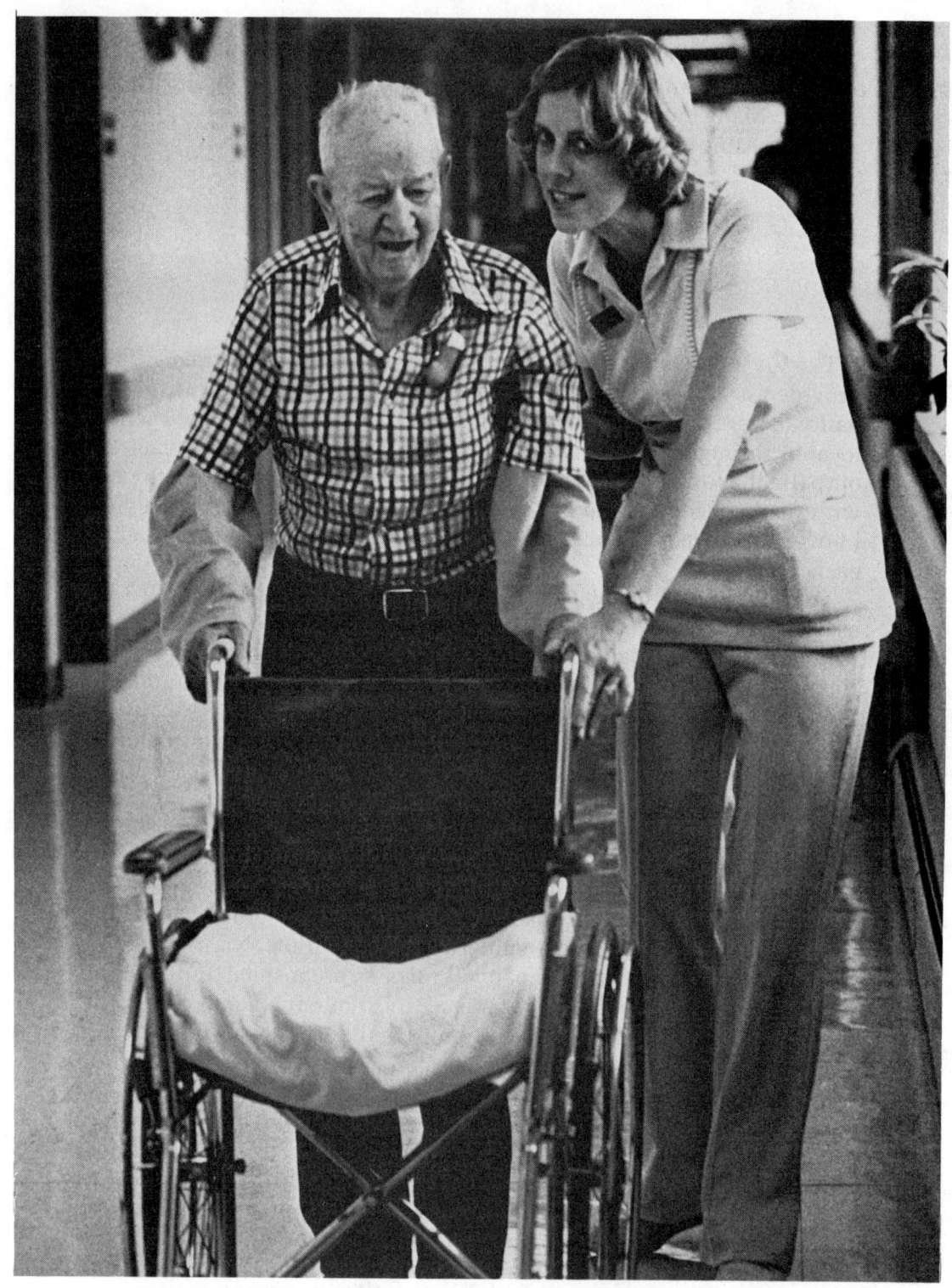

Nurse supports and guides a patient at a VA medical center. (Photo courtesy of the Veterans Administration)

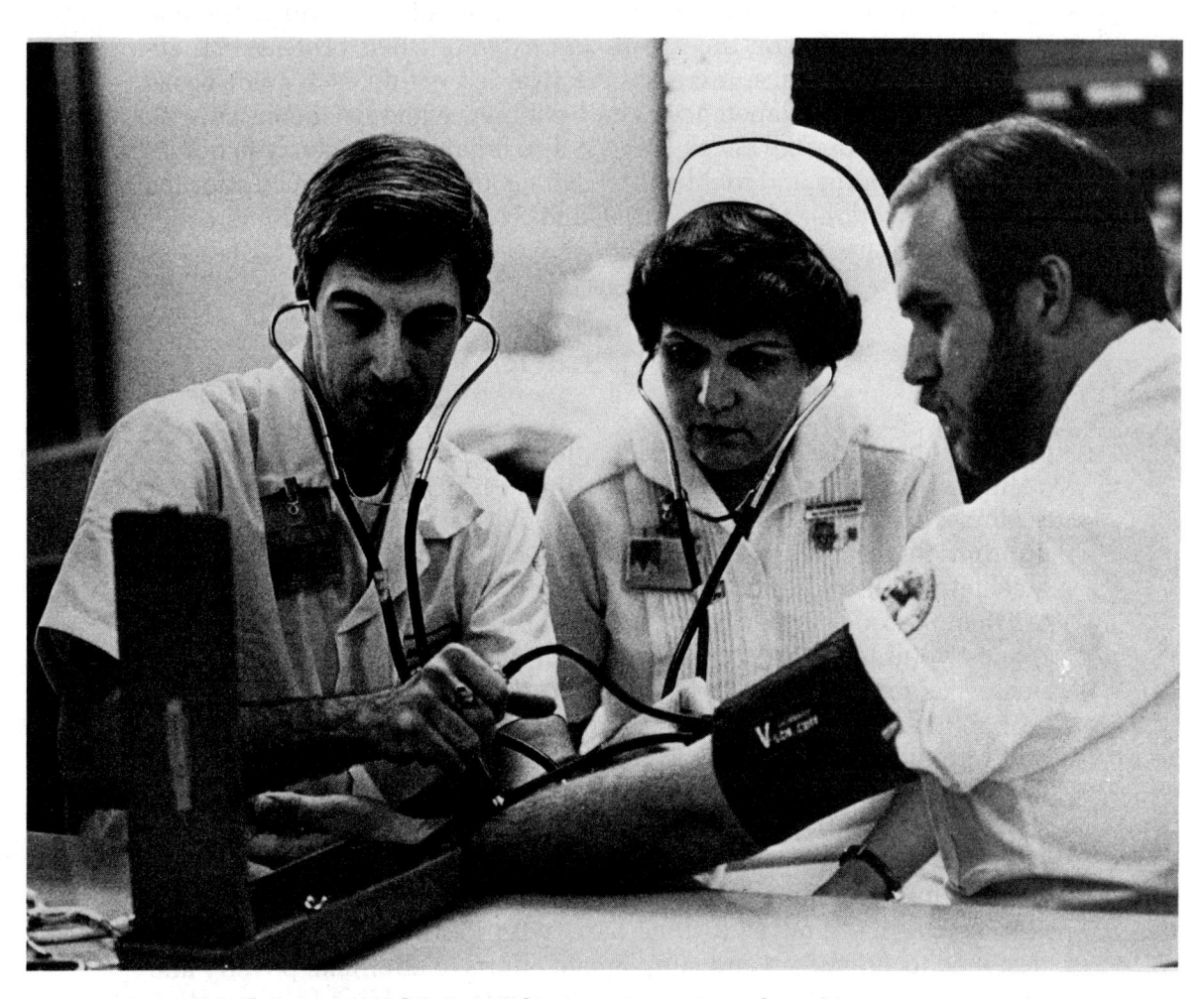

Registered nurse conducting a basic orientation class for nursing assistants in procedures for taking blood tests at a VA medical center. (Photo courtesy of the Veterans Administration)

as respiratory care, coronary care, renal dialysis and other intensive care units. Other courses deal with leadership responsibilities, patient care management and health care administration. Through a program of professional development, career VA nurses can advance to leadership positions in administration, education or research.

Employee benefits and salary for nurses in the VA are good. Benefits include 26 days of vacation, sick leave, national holidays, health insurance in which the Federal government pays part of the premiums, a retirement plan where the VA matches the employee's contribution, credit unions, transfers between medical centers without loss of pay or tenure and tuition assistance for further education.

Salaries for nurses are variable. Nurses are appointed at one of several "grades" depending on the nature and extent of their professional education and experience. Increases are awarded within each grade based on demonstrated competence. The basic pay schedule increases with general federal pay advances. The VA also offers premium pay to nurses who work evening and night shifts. Extra compensation is also afforded those who work holidays, overtime and Sundays, or who are on call.

Peace Corps and VISTA

Nurses have also enjoyed challenging and rewarding experiences in volunteer programs administered by the Peace Corps and VISTA.

Nurses in the Peace Corps receive 9 to 14 weeks of training in the appropriate local language and the cross-cultural skills needed to enter a society with traditions and attitudes different from their own. They are then placed overseas in countries whose needs are critical, and who request volunteers to aid in their economic and social development. The nurses serve for a period of two years, living among the people with whom they work. They are expected to become a part of the community and through their voluntary service demonstrate that people can be an important impetus for change. Currently volunteers, many of them nurses, serve in 63 countries throughout Latin America, Africa, the Near East, Asia and the Pacific.

Other nurses volunteer as VISTA (Volunteers in Service to America) workers, working on a full-time basis with locally sponsored projects designed to strengthen and supplement efforts to eliminate poverty and the related human, social and environmental problems in our nation and its territories. Following a training period these nurses serve for one year by living and working among the needy in urban ghettos, in impoverished small towns and in rural areas such as Appalachia—with migrant workers, on Indian reservations and in institutions for the mentally ill or handicapped.

Nursing During War—One Nurse's Experience

In situations of war, nurses have always made significant contributions. The recent Middle East wars have been no exception. One Lebanese nurse studying in the United States for her master's degree in

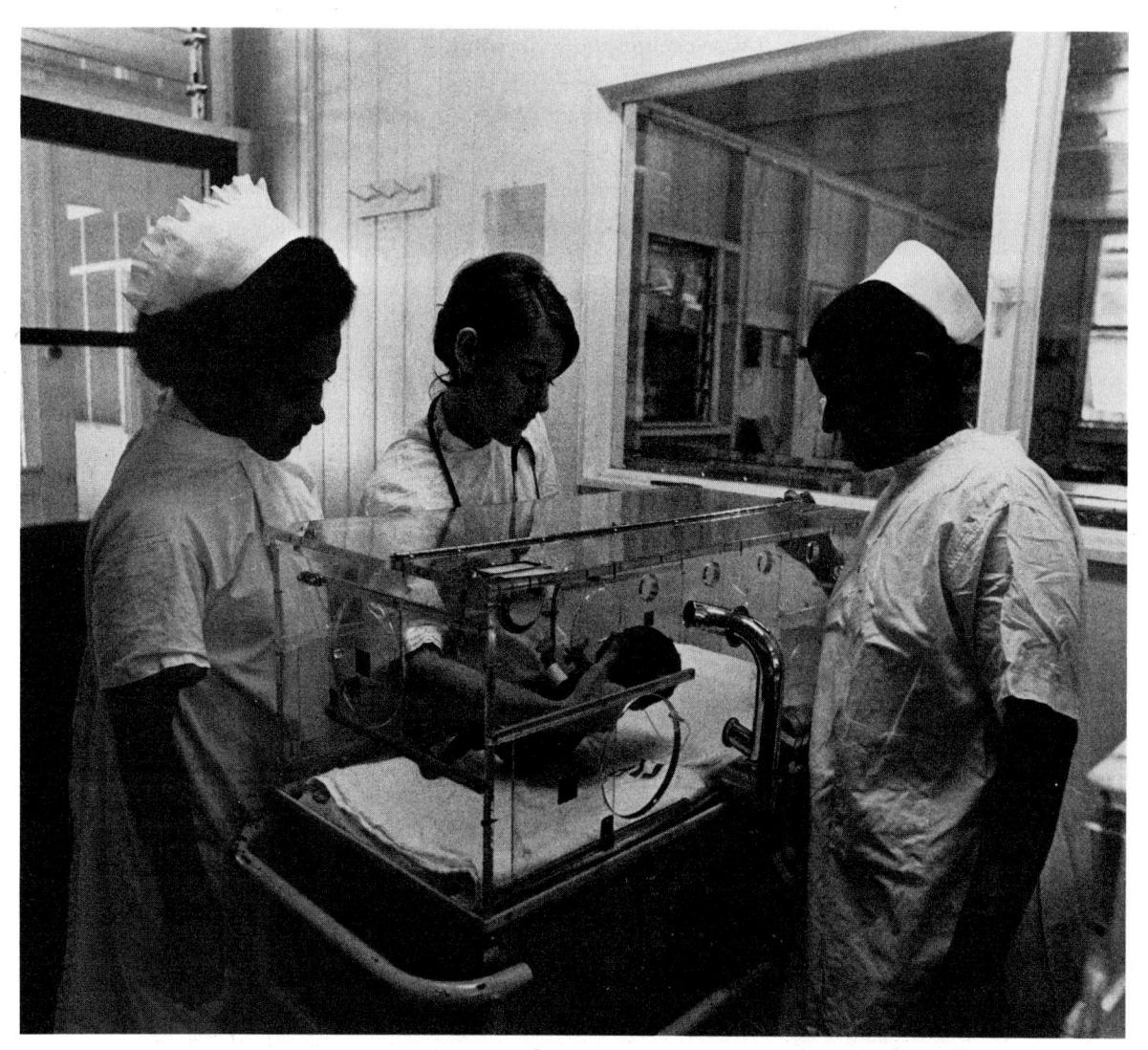

Peace Corps nurse teaching pediatrics to nurses at a hospital in Fiji.
(Photo courtesy of the Peace Corps)

nursing returned to her own country just prior to Israel's attempt to drive the PLO from Beirut. Communicating with her nursing colleagues in the United States she described some of her experiences.

> In February of 1982 she was in charge of the critical care areas of one hospital in Beirut and was also working in another local hospital helping to organize their nursing service. The shooting during that period was sporadic, she commented, and she and her staff got used to it.
> A few months later the situation became unbearable, one she and her nursing colleagues had never been through in their lifetime. She found it difficult to tolerate the stress, the air raids,

shelling, no fruit, vegetables, eggs, water or electricity. Many medical and nursing staff left the city or country with their families. Those that remained worked long and hard. For many weeks she worked from 6 A.M. to 1 A.M. and in an effort to keep up with the wounded she and the nursing staff trained volunteers to help with patient care. At one point in the fighting the hospital was hit and patients fled to the basement where she finally found them. Fortunately no one was hurt in that incident.

At the height of the fighting an average of 200 patients a day were treated in the emergency room. She found the patients burned from the phosphorus bombs the most difficult to care for, both physically and from the standpoint of her emotions. Since tub baths for these burn patients were a priority, the staff used the little fuel they had to warm the bath water for the patients. She and the other nurses had not had a warm tub bath for three months during the fighting.

After the Palestinians had left Beirut and the crisis had eased, she had an opportunity to think and reflect. Commenting to American nursing friends about the role nursing had played, she noted that during the crisis it was nursing that kept the hospital going. It was the nursing staff who cared for patients over 24 hours, supported them and listened to their complaints despite the nurses' own miserable working conditions. It was an experience she will long remember.

For Further Information

Write:

Action/Peace Corps
Office of Recruitment
Washington, DC 20525

Air Force Nurse Corps
HQ USAF/SGN
Bolling Air Force Base
Washington, DC 20332

Army Nurse Corps
Office of the Surgeon General
Department of the Army
Washington, DC 20310

Indian Health Service
Nursing Services Branch
5600 Fishers Lane
Rockville, MD 20857

Navy Nurse Corps
Nurse Corps Division
Bureau of Medicine and Surgery
Navy Department
Washington, DC 20372

Veterans Administration
810 Vermont Avenue, N.W.
Washington, DC 20420

Read:

Health Care Services for Native Americans.
   American Nurses Association
   Publication No. M-28

The Indian Health Program.
   U.S. Department of Health and Human Services
   DHHS Publication No. (HSA) 80-1003, 1980.

Leininger, M. "Transcultural Nursing: Its Progress and Its Future." *Nursing and Health Care* 2:365, 1981.

Masson, V. *International Nursing.* New York: Springer, 1981.

"Nurses Needed in Armed Forces, Says Brig. General Hazel Johnson." *The American Nurse* 14:20, 1982.

Nurse Careers in the Veterans Administration.
   Government Publication No. IB-10-11, March 1980.

Parsons, M. and DeLoor, R. "The Veterans Administration Today." *Nursing and Health Care* 3:126, 1982.

Redding, S. "Peace Corps Volunteer in Africa." *International Nursing* by VeNeta Masson. New York: Springer, 1981.

7.

Education, Research, and Combined Careers

In addition to the many careers possible in nursing practice, exciting careers are also possible in nursing education, nursing research and in careers which combine nursing with fields such as law, business and industry.

Nurse Educators

Good nurse educators are nurses who have an excellent understanding of practice problems. They are usually people who enjoy teaching students as much as they enjoy practicing nursing.

Positions for nurse educators are available in practical, diploma, associate, baccalaureate, master's and doctoral degree programs in nursing. The focus of each of the types of nursing programs is different, as is the type and level of student and the preparation needed to teach in each of the programs.

Practical Nursing Education

As previously described, educational programs to prepare practical nurses are one full year in length and include a few basic science courses as well as nursing courses. The educational programs are often based in hospitals, in private vocational schools, and in some public high schools. The classes are taught by nursing faculty and are usually attended only by the practical nursing students.

Faculty teaching in programs for practical nursing are generally expected to work a 40-hour week. They usually have a 12-month contract with one month's paid vacation in addition to paid sick leave and standard holidays. Faculty are also responsible for attending committee meetings within the school, for counseling students and for attending nursing meetings in the nursing community.

> An instructor in a school of practical nursing described her work. Her work day was either spent in a hospital, supervising students giving care to patients, or teaching classes at the school of nursing. Since the focus of practical nursing is on having the graduate provide bedside care, the majority of her time was spent in the clinical setting from 6:30 A.M. until 3:30 P.M. Her day in the clinical setting was similar to that described in the following section by a diploma school instructor, except that this instructor for practical nurses had no office space in the hospital. Her office was located in the school of nursing, several blocks away.
>
> Classes began at 8:30 A.M. and consisted of anatomy and physiology, growth and development, family, and fundamentals of nursing, all taught by the nursing faculty. Following these classes were classes in specialty areas of nursing: medical surgical, obstetrics and pediatrics, with clinical experience in each of these areas. (She taught fundamentals of nursing, obstetrics and pediatrics and participated in teaching the courses on growth and development and the family.) The students she taught ranged from 17 to 55 years of age. She taught women from a wide variety of backgrounds who were taking on a new role and acquiring a marketable skill.
>
> The most satisfying aspect of the work identified by faculty is seeing the students develop good bedside nursing skills. The two frustrations most commonly cited by the registered nursing faculty were deficient academic preparation of students who entered the programs and the frustration of not being able to teach a role that is not one's own.

The minimum educational requirement for teaching in a school of practical nursing is usually a B.S.N. Advancement comes with a master's degree, which would qualify an individual for an administrative role, e.g., director of a school of practical nursing.

CHARACTERISTICS IMPORTANT FOR THIS TYPE OF WORK INCLUDE:

- interest in teaching
- patience and the ability to work with beginning students

- interest in bedside patient teaching
- commitment to practical nursing

Diploma Nursing Education

As described in chapter 1, diploma nursing is hospital-based education. The educational programs run from 18 to 36 months in length and are taught by nursing faculty hired by the hospital school of nursing. Faculty from colleges or medical schools may be hired to teach specific courses, such as anatomy and physiology. Nursing students are usually the only students who attend these classes, although sometimes a school may make arrangements with a nearby college so students can take courses there.

Nursing faculty teaching in diploma schools may teach classroom content in nursing practice, such as pediatric nursing or surgical nursing, and supervise students in caring for patients with problems in these areas in a hospital associated with the school. Faculty are also responsible for participating in school committees, such as curriculum, student evaluation and faculty development. The faculty may also serve on nursing committees in the associated hospital.

Faculty members in diploma schools are generally expected to work 40 hours a week. They have a twelve-month contract with one month's paid vacation in addition to paid sick leave and standard holidays. Educational preparation for employment in diploma schools generally ranges from a bachelor's to a master's degree in nursing. There is a national trend toward closing diploma programs. Therefore, the employment opportunities in this area can be expected to decrease.

> An instructor teaching in a diploma nursing program recently described her work. She arrives at the hospital at 7:30 A.M. and goes to her office on the fifth floor. This floor is a 50-bed unit of men and women with medical or surgical disorders, such as uncontrolled diabetes, heart problems and urinary infections. At approximately 7:45 A.M. she checks the students' assignment sheet which she has completed the previous day to see if any of the assigned patients have been discharged, transferred or if their conditions have changed markedly, which might require an adjustment in the assignments. At 8:00 A.M. the morning report begins. All the students are present to receive the night nurse's report on the condition and treatment schedule for each of their assigned patients.
>
> After the morning report the instructor meets briefly with the students, reviews their assignments and shares any special information on the patients that she has learned on previous days.

She then checks to see if students will be performing procedures that were new to them, such as injections, catheterizations or dressing changes. If so, she schedules time to talk with the students, review the procedure and the plan to supervise the student later in carrying it out.

This instructor may have 10 to 12 students in the unit to which she is assigned. Usually eight of these are freshmen and the remainder are seniors who require less direct supervision. The seniors usually need direction and consultation in refining their skills, handling difficult situations and in leading small groups of other students, practical nurses and aides in providing care to a small group of patients.

The instructor stays in the unit the remainder of the day, periodically checking the students to see that all is progressing well with their patient care assignments. She also spends time in her office in the unit, working on such things as lectures, reports, committee assignments and student evaluations. Several days a week the freshmen leave the unit at 1 P.M. for class. If it is a class the instructor teaches, she too leaves and another instructor from a nearby unit drops by periodically to assist the remaining students with any new procedures or with any problems that have occurred.

Shortly before 4 P.M. the instructor checks which students will be in the unit the following day and schedules the patient assignments. She tries to plan these assignments so that students have an opportunity to acquire necessary learning experiences, while at the same time matching the students' present abilities with the complexity of the care the patients require.

Nursing faculty teaching in diploma programs have cited the ability to provide some direct patient care, see young people become bedside nurses, and good salaries as satisfactions of their jobs. They say frustrations of the work include the demands of staff nurses to have students perform routine tasks during their time in the units rather than those that provide new learning experiences, comparisons of past diploma education to the current program, and difficulty instituting educational changes.

CHARACTERISTICS IMPORTANT FOR THIS TYPE OF WORK INCLUDE:

- interest in teaching and development of students
- interest in hospital nursing
- clinical expertise
- commitment to diploma nursing education

Collegiate Programs

Faculty in collegiate nursing programs, whether they are for associate, baccalaureate, master's or doctoral degrees, generally have flexible working hours. Instructors are expected to teach, supervise and be available to advise students, and participate in committees and the work of the college and university. Faculty are free to schedule their time around these responsibilities. Collegiate nursing faculty usually have 9- or 10-month teaching contracts, and are off on usual holidays and during student vacation periods. Educational preparation for employment in collegiate nursing programs generally ranges from post-baccalaureate to doctoral preparation in nursing, or an associated discipline depending on the level of instruction. In general, if you are thinking about a career in academe, you should assume that a master's degree in nursing will be the minimum educational credential. For maximum career mobility, a doctoral degree is desirable and may become mandatory in the future to achieve professorial rank.

Associate Degree Nursing Education

Associate degree nursing programs are based in community colleges and in four-year colleges and universities that grant associate degrees. Since nursing students in these programs are students in the college, they take arts and science courses with other students in the institution. Nursing courses are taught by nursing faculty hired by the nursing school or department.

Nursing faculty teach nursing content in the classroom and supervise students in caring for patients in many types of settings. These settings may include community hospitals, nursing homes, clinics, nursery schools and community agencies.

Faculty are responsible for participating in nursing committees in the department or school, such as curriculum and faculty development. They are also expected to participate with other schools or departments on committees that deal with academic issues that involve personnel policies, long-range planning, and promotion and tenure.

> A faculty member who has a position in an associate degree program in a private institution described her work in the following way.
>
> Because the college has no hospital directly affiliated with it, on the two days she supervises students in their clinical practice, she drives 30 miles to the hospital. She also drives to the hospital the day prior to the students' experience in order

to make out their patient assignments. Of course, this is not necessarily the case for all such faculty members as many live nearer to the clinical facility. The two days of clinical experience for students in the hospital are similar to those previously described by the diploma faculty member. The instructor arrives at the unit prior to the 8 A.M. morning report and updates the student assignments. Following the morning report she meets briefly with the students and reviews their assignments and any new procedures they may need to perform. She spends the remainder of the day in the hospital helping and working with the students. She rarely brings committee work or other paperwork with her to the hospital, since she has no office there. Much of her spare time in the unit is spent doing public relations, such as talking with or helping out the nursing staff because the instructor and students are considered "guests" in the hospital. During one semester, two additional schools had students in this particular unit, although not on the same days. This required considerable work and coordination of effort with the staff of both the unit and the other schools.

During the three days she spends at the college, she teaches a three-hour class from 9 A.M. to 12 P.M. on two of those days. In the afternoons she prepares for the next class, corrects student assignments, does committee assignments, or attends department or college meetings. On Fridays she has neither class nor clinical supervision and may choose to work in her office at the college or at home. She may choose to take the day off, knowing that if she does, work may still have to be done on the weekend.

This flexibility in work schedules, working with other knowledgeable faculty within a college setting and seeing students succeed and develop in their career are satisfactions cited often by faculty teaching in associate degree programs. Frustrations mentioned include not having enough clinical time to teach all that they want to students, and a desire for greater control of the college's entrance requirements for nursing students.

CHARACTERISTICS IMPORTANT FOR THIS TYPE OF WORK INCLUDE:

- interest in teaching and development of students
- ability to negotiate clinical problems
- flexibility
- clinical expertise

Baccalaureate Degree Nursing Education

Baccalaureate degree nursing programs are based in four-year colleges and universities. Nursing students take arts and science courses with other students in the university or college. Their nursing courses are taught by faculty in the nursing department or school.

Nursing faculty in baccalaureate nursing programs teach nursing in the classroom and supervise students in a variety of clinical settings one or more days a week. The non-hospital settings in which students have experience are generally greater in baccalaureate programs as compared to associate degree programs. Faculty in these programs are expected to participate in school, department and college or university committees. They are also usually expected to participate in nursing organizations on the local and perhaps state and national level. Research, publication and the presentation of papers at state and national meetings may be required for promotion and tenure.

While faculty teaching in undergraduate nursing programs may have a number of older students in their classes, the majority of students are from 18 to 22 years old. Faculty spend considerable time counseling and advising undergraduate students, since they often need much direction in beginning their careers. Many students in this age group are experiencing the personal turbulence of their late teens and need the additional help of mature instructors to guide them. Faculty teaching in graduate programs often have an almost peer relationship with graduate students, who usually have defined their career goals. Faculty then serve as resources and mentors to these students.

A faculty member teaching in a private university baccalaureate nursing program shared her teaching experience with us.

> She too spends two days each week supervising students in a clinical setting. But she spends the remaining three days a week teaching class and carrying out faculty responsibilities at the university. The school is affiliated with a nearby hospital and so she simply walks two blocks from her office to the hospital unit where she supervises students. The unit is the inpatient psychiatric unit for the local community mental health center. She arrives at the unit at approximately 7:45 A.M. and checks with the night staff about the general behavior of the patients that the students will be working with. If there have been any behavioral problems or significant changes in patients' conditions, she communicates these to the incoming students.
>
> Students arrive at the unit by at least 8 A.M. and help or supervise two patients in bathing and dressing. They will work with these same patients for the entire semester. Breakfast ar-

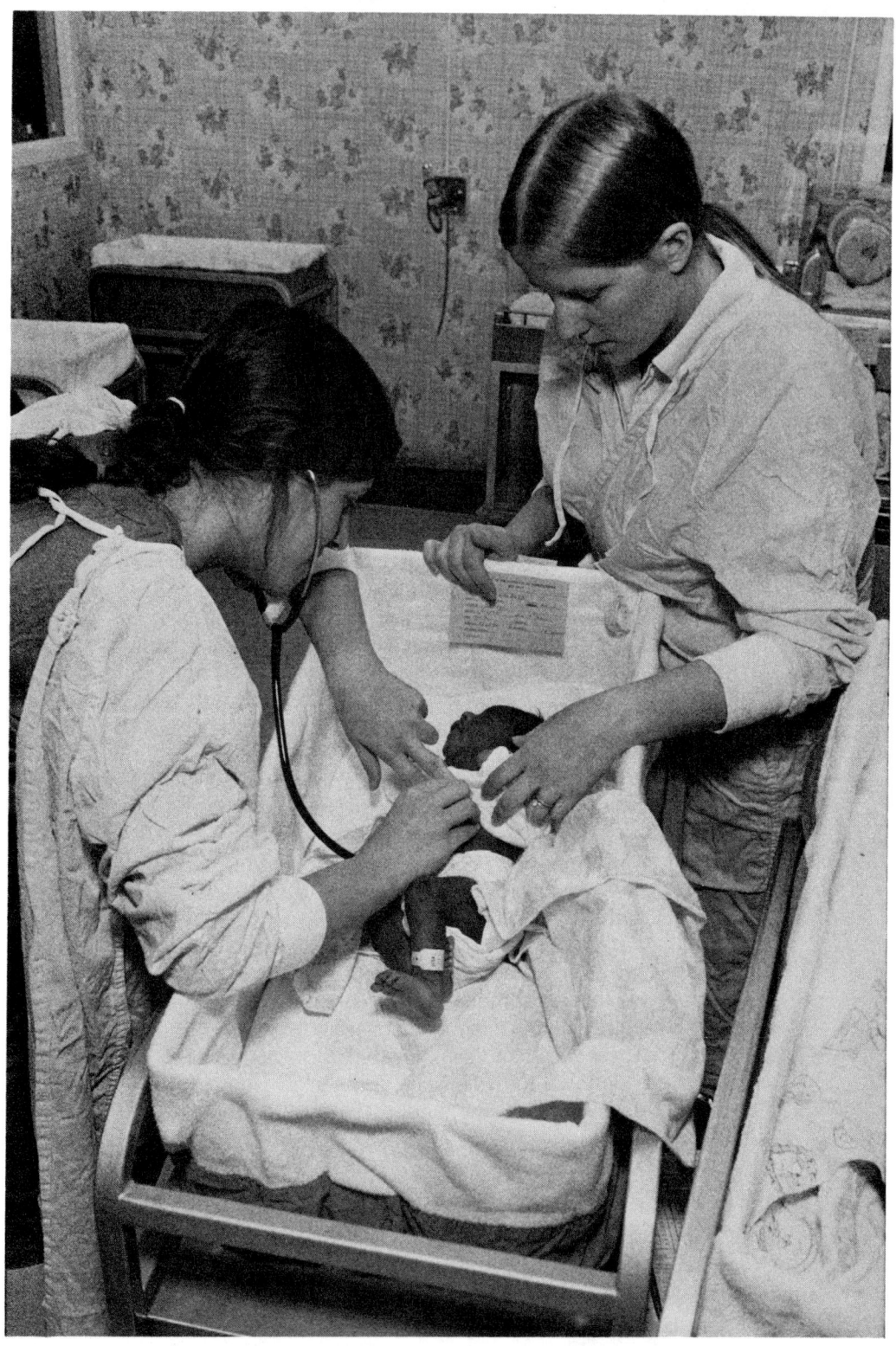

Supervising a student in assessment of a newborn.

rives about 8:15 and students may sit and have coffee with their patients or excuse themselves to listen to the taped report on patients prepared by the night nursing staff, if they have not already done so. The tape serves the same purpose as the morning report described previously. They also talk with the primary nurse about the patients' progress and schedule for the day.

The nursing faculty member meets with each student following breakfast and discusses the patients' schedule and the students' plans for working with the patients during the day. She also collects written assignments called process recordings from each student. These assignments are recordings of 15 to 20 minutes of conversation between the student and patient which are intended to help the students analyze and improve their communication techniques.

Since the unit is small, most activity occurs in the day room, where the instructor spends the next several hours participating in patient-student activities. She also checks with the head nurse, the recreational therapist, physician and social worker to determine if there are additional activities planned for the day in which students might participate. This often includes group therapy sessions, court hearings for patients, outings in the community for select patients or meetings with a patient's family and some members of the health care team. Usually, the staff keeps the instructor informed of any activities that would be interesting or helpful to students. This faculty member says she has had several groups of nursing students in this unit for the past few years and the working relationships have been very good. Some of her former students are now staff nurses in the unit.

Three times during the day, at 10 A.M., noon and 2 P.M., she supervises one student giving medications to all patients on the unit. Periodically throughout the day she walks about the unit talking with patients and helping students work with patients who may be especially hostile, depressed or withdrawn. Around 3 P.M., the faculty member, the students and any staff members who are able to attend meet together. Students discuss and analyze their work, and seek feedback, comments or suggestions from fellow students, staff and the nursing faculty. Following this conference, the students report off to their patients' primary nurse.

Faculty teaching in baccalaureate nursing programs say that seeing the students develop in their careers, and the shared collegiality among nursing faculty and the faculties of other disciplines within the college or university are satisfactions of their work. Frustrations often cited include lack of time to pursue writing and research, and too much time spent in committee meetings.

CHARACTERISTICS IMPORTANT FOR THIS TYPE OF WORK INCLUDE:

- interest in teaching and development of students
- clinical expertise
- flexibility

Master's Degree Nursing Education

Master's degree programs in nursing are found in university settings. They prepare nurses to function in expanded nursing roles in a variety of clinical specialties such as pediatrics, midwifery and psychiatric nursing. Some programs also offer preparation for teaching and administrative roles in nursing.

Faculty in master's programs teach nursing in the classroom and in the clinical setting. In the clinical setting, faculty may serve as resources or consultants to master's students or may supervise students' practice as they learn new skills or nursing techniques. Faculty are also expected to participate in department, school and university committees and activities, professional organizational activities and community service activities. Student recruitment may also be an important function of graduate faculty. Faculty who teach in master's programs are usually expected to carry out research and to publish.

A faculty member teaching in a master's degree nursing program described her schedule in the following way.

> Monday is a "workday" spent in faculty, university or school committee meetings or in preparing work for them. It is also a time to carry out other work such as making student evaluations, correcting assignments, negotiating agreements with clinical agencies, preparing tests and interviewing prospective students. On Tuesday she teaches a graduate class from 9 A.M. to 12 noon in high risk childbearing. Every Wednesday from 8 A.M. to 4 P.M. she is in the hospital working with graduate students to improve their skills. Unlike undergraduate supervision, however, she serves mainly as a resource and consultant to the students, who are already registered nurses. While in the hospital, she may have students in several units. She moves from unit to unit, periodically spending time with each student to help them with particular clinical problems or specific ap-

proaches to a difficult patient situation. Very often she helps students give direct patient care in order to demonstrate a particular technique.

Since the students have clinical experience in a variety of agencies throughout the region and are supervised by master's prepared nurses in those agencies, she spends Thursday mornings visiting the agencies and consulting on the students' progress. On Thursday afternoon she leads a two-hour clinical seminar in which the students discuss the work they have done with patients during the week.

Friday is spent on research and writing projects expected of graduate faculty. In addition to completing several articles this year, she is under contract to write a textbook. While some Fridays are spent in the library, this faculty member says she often spends Fridays working at home where interruptions are fewer. Very often her work carries over to the weekend.

Graduate nursing faculty have cited the intellectual stimulation and challenge of working with graduate nursing students and faculty in other disciplines within the university as satisfactions of this type of work. Frustrating aspects often mentioned are the lack of adequate time during the week for research and writing, and the high expectations for promotion and tenure.

CHARACTERISTICS IMPORTANT FOR THIS TYPE OF WORK INCLUDE:

- interest in teaching and development of students
- intellectual curiosity and interest in research
- ability to organize time and resources

Doctoral Degree Nursing Education

Doctoral degree programs are located in major universities. They prepare researchers and people in nursing who aspire to become professors, deans and high level executors in the health care industry. Faculty teach advanced courses in nursing theory, research and sometimes clinical practice. They also direct doctoral students in carrying out their thesis requirements. They must participate in the work of the university, as well as in the school or department with which they are associated.

Education, Research, and Combined Careers   145

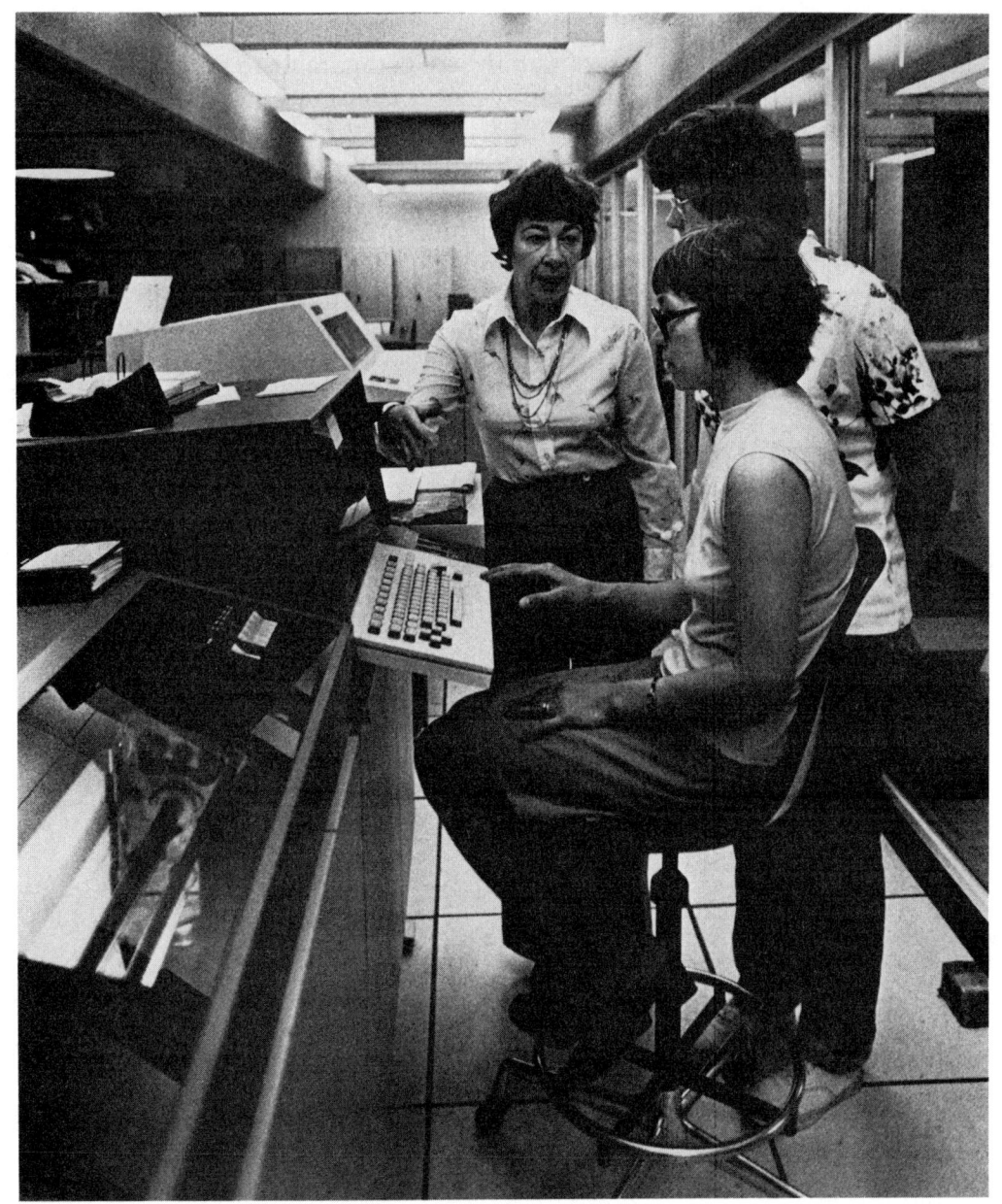

Doctoral students learn about computers.

Faculty teaching in doctoral programs are expected to be leaders in the profession, as demonstrated by presenting papers at the national level, carrying out research and publishing their work.

Faculties in collegiate schools of nursing generally advance their careers through research, publications, presentation of papers, teaching excellence and their ability to develop projects that attract outside funding. Some faculty pursue administrative positions such as department heads, and deanships.

Faculty salaries in schools of nursing are comparable to those in other disciplines within the college or university. They are generally less than those of nurses in administrative positions within hospitals or health care agencies who have the same credentials and who are on a twelve-month contract. But many faculty prefer the flexibility their schedules allow them to the pay differential of nursing service administrators. Many are also able to draw considerable additional income from royalties, consultant fees and honoraria that come from the outside activities they must be involved in to advance their careers.

CHARACTERISTICS IMPORTANT FOR THIS TYPE OF WORK INCLUDE:

- interest in students and teaching
- good communication skills
- interest in developing others
- ability to work with groups
- leadership skills

Educational Administration

The role of the dean in a school of nursing is very demanding and requires much maturity, political astuteness and sophistication. Most deans have come up through the academic ranks and are also tenured professors.

Deans have the ultimate responsibility for determining the direction their schools and educational programs will take through democratic leadership. At the same time, they must remain up-to-date and see to it that the faculty does so as well. Deans must be excellent managers because they are usually responsible for maintaining the fiscal soundness of the school and supervising large support staffs of secretaries, admission and record clerks, business managers, recruiters and administration assistants. In large schools, the dean may employ associate and assistant deans to assume a share of their academic work.

In addition, the work of deans extends far beyond the borders of their schools and five eight-hour days. They must meet with the deans of

Education, Research, and Combined Careers

other schools in the university and with the chief administration officers, such as the president, vice-presidents, provost and financial officers. At these meetings the dean must be able to communicate clearly the strengths and needs of the school and the profession. Often, deans are members of the boards of corporations and foundations. They must know state and national officials and serve on national high-level policy committees in and out of the profession. There are also many social events that must be attended to keep up professional contacts and to maintain the visibility of the school. Frequently, these contacts may spell the difference between successfully obtaining financial support for the school from endowments and grants or going without it.

Deans say the most rewarding part of their job is working with faculty and colleagues to promote the excellence of the school and the profession. The most difficult part is maintaining sufficient energy to meet the taxing demands of their position.

CHARACTERISTICS IMPORTANT FOR THIS TYPE OF WORK INCLUDE:

- assertiveness
- management skills
- energy
- dedication to education and the profession
- ability to set priorities

Nursing Research

While careers in nursing research are still somewhat limited, opportunities in the field are increasing. Nurses may be employed in departments of nursing research in large hospitals. The aim of these departments is usually to help nurses within that setting carry out research focused on improving patient care. Many more nurses are involved in research in academic settings where they conduct a variety of investigations into theoretical and clinical problems. Nursing research in these settings is essential to the development and quality of graduate education in nursing as well as to improvement of patient care.

Two current lines of investigation by nurse researchers illustrate the impact of clinical research in nursing on improvements in patient care.

Research on the formulas of stomach tube feedings used by many cancer patients, the effects of its temperature and the time it takes to be transported through the digestive tract are the interests of several groups of nurse researchers headed by Barbara Hansen, Ph.D., RN. One of the groups' many findings thus far has shown that many patients maintained on stomach tube feedings show a lactose (sugar) intolerance not evident when they eat normal diets. While on routine stomach feedings these same patients experience stomach discomfort, nausea and severe diarrhea. As a result of the groups' work, at least one manufacturer of the tube feeding formulas has changed its preparation to eliminate the lactose base.

The research of several other nurses has important implications for the prevention of areas of intestinal destruction in premature infants.

In 1976, two nurses, Carol Measel and Gene Anderson, noted that restless premature infants developing intestinal distention would become relaxed and could be tubefed successfully if allowed to suck on a pacifier during and following each feeding. Their study of 59 premature infants assigned to treatment and control groups showed that treated infants were ready for bottle feeding three and one-half days earlier and therefore required 27 fewer tube feedings. The infants gained weight faster and were discharged from the hospital an average of four days sooner.

Their research has been reproduced and extended twice. In one study Dr. Anderson collaborated with a group of developmental psychologists. Their findings were essentially the same regarding weight gain and infant readiness for bottle feeding. Additionally, the 30 treated infants went home eight days sooner than the controls, resulting in cost savings of over $100,000. The second extension of their work was conducted by a pediatrician and her associates. Their findings regarding infant weight gain, earlier bottle feeding, earlier discharge and increased weight gain were similar to the earlier nursing studies. The results of the work by these nurse researchers have important implications for preventing intestinal complications and subsequent major surgery in this group of small premature infants.*

Currently there are numerous other lines of investigation being pursued by nurse researchers. Some of these include the physiological effects on the mother and fetus of anxiety during labor, developmental

---

*Measel, C. and Anderson, S. "Non-nutritive Sucking During Tube Feedings: Effect Upon Clinical Course in Premature Infants." *Journal of Obstetric and Neonatal Nursing* 8:265, 1979.

effects of early infant stimulation, differences in temperament of very low birthweight babies, the effects of health beliefs on how people maintain their health and how preoperation teaching should be done.

Conducting Research

Investigators often face the dilemma of whether to conduct research only if funds are available or to go ahead even if they are not. The issues to be considered vary—working on a particular topic may be considered important by funding agencies, there may be big cutbacks in government or foundation research budgets, data may be available at the time and research cannot wait for a grant to be processed, or a researcher may not yet have established a reputation for conducting research.

Some nurses wait to secure funding for their study because the equipment or supplies needed to begin require funding. Other nurse researchers begin without money. Lynda Holmstrom, a sociologist, and Ann Burgess, a psychiatric nurse, began their work investigating the effects of rape on victims in 1972, and shared some of their experiences conducting research without funding.

> In 1972 little scholarly research existed on the problems rape victims experienced and few clinical services were available to help them. The goals of their study were to investigate the problems of victims and to provide counseling services to them.
>
> They began their study after getting the cooperation of the nursing service of a large urban hospital. Although they submitted grant proposals to several agencies, they were not funded. One agency, a foundation supporting research in women's studies, told them their proposal was well written but that the agency was not interested in rape.
>
> Although the two were full-time faculty members, one in a college and the other in a university, they were committed to the research. During a period of one year they interviewed 146 rape victims. As Holmstrom and Burgess comment, conducting interviews at the hospital when rape victims were admitted was easily arranged. Most victims came to the hospital at times that did not overlap with their teaching responsibilities. Child victims usually arrived in late afternoon or early evening while adult victims arrived in the middle of the night. Both investigators saw each victim.
>
> In addition to being interviewed on admission to the emergency room, the investigators conducted weekly follow-up interviews, usually by telephone, based on the victim's emotional

problems. Telephone calls were fit in between their faculty commitments. If the rape victims decided to press charges, one of the interviewers accompanied the victim to court. The investigators found that observing in court was difficult to manage. Court delays were numerous. Many times victims went to court to find that their case had been postponed and rescheduled at the last minute. Observing during the rape trials and associated courthouse proceedings often took several days. Victims often went to the courthouse a day or two prior to the trial to talk with a district attorney in order to prepare the case. The trials often lasted two to four days. At least one of the researchers attended 22 of the 28 hearings and 10 of the 12 trials. Some court sessions were missed due to conflicting teaching schedules. Finding that they needed additional help supplementing their observations at court and in victims' homes, they incorporated nursing, pre-law, law, political science, psychology and sociology students into their study on a voluntary basis. The nursing students, they found, had an advantage because their public image gave them entree to the victims' homes. Nurses too, were already trained observers, attuned to physical and social aspects of people's lives.*

Prior to the work of Holmstrom and Burgess, little research existed in crisis intervention with rape victims. Their data was used to develop new skills for working with this previously neglected group of patients.

Another team of four faculty investigators shared their experiences in carrying out research with the aid of several small grants. As they noted, having grant money allows you to buy time, by having another faculty member hired to release you from teaching, or by hiring a research assistant to collect the data.

This group of four has just completed a study on ways to reduce breast pain and swelling in new mothers who choose not to breast feed their infants. They are currently collecting data on the effects of a mother's diet on a newborn's chances of becoming jaundiced shortly after birth. Three of the four have just received funding for an additional study investigating earlier hospital discharge of premature infants. The fourth member of the team will be completing requirements for her doctoral degree in the next year. Two of the four faculty work full time while the remaining two are part-time faculty members with full-time family responsibilities involving very young children. Because of their teaching and family commitments, the group

---

*Holstrom, L. and Burgess, A. "Low Cost Research: A Project on a Shoestring." *Nursing Research* 31:123, 1982.

chose to use their monies to hire a research assistant to collect the data for their studies. The group also explained why they chose to conduct research as a group.

By working together, this team is able to work on more than one study at a time; when emergencies arise, usually one of the group is available to handle the crisis; and working together has increased the camaraderie and provided a supportive working group.

The doctorally prepared member of the group has been the principal investigator or team leader on the studies. Because the group has hired a research assistant to collect the study data, she has maintained her full-time faculty responsibilities. At least one-half day each week she reviews the data that has been collected thus far and monitors the progress of the study. She schedules meetings from once a week to once a month with the research team (depending upon the stage and progress of the study) to review and update the team on the findings. She also negotiates with other scientists or heads of laboratories to have samples analyzed and to gain access to patients who might want to participate in the study. She purchases the equipment for the study in consultation with the other team members and has the major responsibilities for handling the day-to-day crises that arise during the study.

For example, during one study when a group of physicians questioned its aspects prior to allowing the nurse researchers access to their patients for possible participation, she was responsible for presenting and explaining the study to the doctors. Also, it was her responsibility to locate a portable centrifuge when one was needed to process blood samples prior to their analysis in the laboratory. She also coordinated the collection and transportation of the blood samples when the research assistant was unavailable. In addition, it is her responsibility to monitor the pace and quality of the research assistant's work. To do this she often meets daily with the research assistant to monitor how well the study is going. Additionally, as part of her responsibility for the budget, she handles the paperwork involved in ordering equipment and supplies, billing for laboratory studies, and writing progress reports and final reports required by the funding agencies. When a study has been finished, the team meets to complete the analysis of the data and to prepare a manuscript for publication.

For the type of clinical research this group conducts, funding is required. They, like many other nurse researchers, have sought and received funding from sources such as the American Nurses Foundation of the American Nurses Association; national and local chapters of Sigma Theta Tau, the nursing honor society; the Division of Nursing, Department of Health and Human Services, and from private foundations such as the Robert Wood Johnson Foundation. Other nurse researchers have received support from drug companies, formula companies and private and federal funding sources.

Nurses working in research positions advance their careers through further development of their research skills, by obtaining research funding and through publication. Some become heads of research departments or research centers.

CHARACTERISTICS IMPORTANT FOR THIS TYPE OF WORK INCLUDE:

- interest in research
- curiosity and creativity
- persistence
- ability to analyze ideas
- ability to write

Combined Careers

An increasing number of nurses are combining their careers in nursing with careers in other fields.

Some nurses have combined their nursing preparation with a career in law. Using their nursing background they are especially valuable to law firms in drawing up contracts for medical facilities, group medical practices and in litigation involving medical malpractice and the quality of hospital care.

Other nurses have combined their nursing experience with careers in industry. Some of these nurses work with companies who design and develop medical technology such as fetal monitors, cardiac monitors and various other types of equipment. Using their nursing preparation, they can explain problems that nurses may have in using the equipment to the designers or developers. These nurses may also offer courses to other nurses in hospitals or agencies who purchase the equipment and who will need a working knowledge of how to interpret the information available from the monitor tracings. These nurses may also develop brochures or booklets on how to use the technology.

Some nurses are employed by insurance companies and work within hospitals to monitor the quality of care patients receive. Other nurses are hired to provide rehabilitative services in patients' homes following hospital discharge. This is an effort on the company's part to speed the patients' recovery and return them to the work force or their usual activities as soon as possible.

Other nurses combine careers in nursing with careers in writing and publishing by becoming journal editors or book editors or assistant editors for nursing and health publications.

The Nurse Editor

There are about 50 periodicals published in nursing each year in addition to hundreds of books. The subject matter covers as many different areas as are found in nursing and range from operating room nursing and maternal-child care to research and theory. In most cases, the periodicals are edited by one or more nurses who work full-time or part-time for the publisher. These nurses are directly responsible for choosing the manuscripts that are published in their magazines. Some copyedit manuscripts themselves, but most have a staff to perform this function. Many of the journals they edit have editorial boards and special panels of experts who help them choose material. However, the editor must coordinate these efforts and oversee the production of the publication so that it is current, maintains reader interest and adheres to editorial policy.

Editors are generally specialists in the area covered by their journal. In order to keep current, they visit clinical facilities and attend many meetings and conventions throughout the country. They also use this time to keep in touch with readers, potential authors and other specialists in the field.

Editors who work for book publishers are usually involved in many phases of a book's production. The choices made by editors in a book publishing house are important not only to the financial stability of their company but to their readership, who depend upon the recency and accuracy of a book's information. Editors must be aware of what new trends are in the field and what publications are needed. They also need to know who in the field is likely to be able to author books on special topics or who could suggest such specialists. This means that many editors must travel a great deal to many parts of the country. It is customary for them to help exhibit books at conventions and at other large gatherings of nurses. During the time they are at meetings, they talk to nurse educators and others to ascertain their needs for books for undergraduate and graduate students in specialty areas. Of course, their understanding of the needs of consumers for the company's publications is important for sales.

Usually, prospective authors submit a proposal to the editor who then requests opinions from nursing experts in the area as to its suitability and sales potential. If the book is deemed appropriate for publication, the editor negotiates a contract with the author. Once the contract has been signed, the editor works along with the author or authors to keep the production of the work on schedule.

All editors must spend a good deal of their time with people in various capacities. They see this as both a rewarding and sometimes difficult experience. They all cite the joy of seeing a book or journal arrive on the market as a highpoint in their jobs.

International Consultation

Since Florence Nightingale, who helped to establish the first nursing schools in this country, nurses have traveled across the world to help other nurses improve the care of people. International travel can be exciting, and can take the form of giving seminars, lectures or direct consultation about clinical or employment opportunities offered by organizations such as the International Congress of Nurses or the World Health Organization. Some nurses make visits as part of special seminar groups or individually because of their special expertise in an area.

University of Pennsylvania faculty members have done consultation or given papers in such far-flung places as Kenya, Nigeria, Jordan, Israel, Australia and Brazil; colleagues have also been to China, Russia and Spain.

Usually, the opportunity for international consultation comes only after you are well established in your field. But sometimes it comes about in odd ways. Dr. Dirschel, Dean of the College of Nursing at Seton Hall University, was invited to join Governor Brendan Byrne of New Jersey and his party on a trip to China because his wife did not care for the idea that all the other university officials were men. The trip resulted in an agreement to send two faculty members from the College to the Hangzhow School of Nursing where they will help introduce faculty and students to concepts and techniques used in Western nursing.

Because international consultation is usually of brief duration, you need to be a person who can readily adapt to circumstances that may be very different from those you are accustomed to. Even the best housing in a developing country may not have running water. "Boning up" on the culture is essential before you leave. Jet lag and a strange diet need to be conquered in 24 hours to maintain a clear head. But in spite of it all, you can return home with a memory of experiences no tour guide can provide, since you are among colleagues who have access to many things you might want to see or know about.

Nursing School Recruiter

One nurse who has combined her nursing background with her interest in students and counseling now works in an admission and recruitment office in a school of nursing. In this role she interviews prospective nursing students, organizes and runs programs on the university campus and in high schools to educate students, parents, guidance counselors and the public at large about nursing and the career opportunities in this field.

A typical day for this nurse recruiter includes interviewing undergraduate student applicants, answering telephone calls for information on graduate and undergraduate nursing education, writing articles for brochures or newspapers about nursing, helping students who have already been admitted plan their careers, talking to guidance counselors about nursing and answering letters requesting information about nursing or the school's programs.

This nurse commented that the most satisfying part of her job is the feeling that she is combining her nursing background with other skills she has developed to promote a profession she loves and in this role, being able to bring intelligent, enthusiastic and personable people into nursing. Her major frustration with her work is combating the outdated television stereotype of nursing that much of the public still believes is true. Skills important for success in this type of work include good communication skills, knowledge of and commitment to the profession, salesmanship and a sense of humor.

Combined Teaching and Practice Positions

Some nurses combine a career through joint appointments to a school of nursing and, most frequently, to a hospital or, less frequently, to a community service agency, such as a visiting nurse service. These nurses spend a portion of their time each week or month teaching as a faculty member in a nursing school and the other portion of their time delivering care to patients, functioning in the hospital as a clinical specialist or specialty practitioner.

As nurses function in a joint role, students are able to see that they are able to practice nursing and clearly relate the theory they are teaching into practice. Current trends in education, health care delivery and research can be easily transferred from the educational setting to the practice setting by the nurse in a joint position. In addition, the nurse can function as a liaison between the two settings, identifying resources that are available in one setting that might also be used in the other. These individuals are also able to identify problems in clinical practice that are in need of research. They can also initiate a study, establish a research team from the educational and practice settings or refer problems to a researcher in either setting. Some of the commonly identified problems of working in a joint appointment include a long work week and the possibly decreased chance of receiving tenure at the college or university.

For Further Information

Write:

American Nurses Association
2420 Pershing Road
Kansas City, MO 64108

Council of Nurse Researchers
American Nurses Association
2420 Pershing Road
Kansas City, MO 64108

National League for Nursing
10 Columbus Circle
New York, NY 10019

Midwest Alliance in Nursing
Room 108-BR
Indiana University
1100 West Michigan Street
Indianapolis, IN 46223

New England Board of Higher Education
School Street
Wenham, MA 01984

Southern Regional Education Board
1340 Spring Street, N.W.
Atlanta, GA 30309

Western Interstate Commission for
    Higher Education
P.O. Drawer P
Boulder, CO 80302

Sigma Theta Tau
1100 West Michigan Street
Indianapolis, IN 46223

The Robert Wood Johnson Foundation
P.O. Box 2316
Princeton, NJ 08540

National Institute of Health
9000 Rockville Pike
Bethesda, MD 20205

Read:

Abstracts of ANF Funded Research 1979–1980.
American Nurses Association
Publication No. FD-26

Associate Degree Education for Nursing 1979–80.
National League for Nursing
Publication No. 23-1309

Baccalaureate Education in Nursing: Key to a Professional Career in Nursing 1979–80.
National League for Nursing
Publication No. 15-1311

Blazeck, A.; Selekman, J.; Timpe, M.; and Wolf, Z. "Unification: Nursing Education and Nursing Practice." Nursing and Health Care 3:18, 1982.

A Case for Baccalaureate Preparation in Nursing.
American Nurses Association
Publication No. NE-6

College Teaching: Putting the Pieces Together.
National League for Nursing
Publication No. 23-1792

Concepts and Components of Effective Teaching.
National League for Nursing
Publication No. 16-1750

Dirschel, K. "Teaching Nursing in China—An Exchange Program." Nursing Outlook 29:722, 1981.

Education for Nursing: The Diploma Way 1979–80.
National League for Nursing
Publication No. 16-1314

Entry into Nursing Practice.
American Nurses Association
Publication No. NE-4

Esler, R. "Getting a New Job." *American Journal of Nursing* 81:758, 1981.

Guidelines for the Investigative Function of Nurses. American Nurses Association
Publication No. D-69

Master's Education in Nursing: Route to Opportunities in Contemporary Nursing 1979–80.
National League for Nursing
Publication No. 15-1312

Nursing Research: Synopses of Selected Clinical Studies.
American Nurses Association
Publication No. D-67

Pilous, B. "Advantages of Part Time Nursing." *The AJN Guide.* New York: American Journal of Nursing Company, 1982.

Practical Nursing Career-1980.
National League for Nursing
Publication No. 38-1328

Research Priorities for the 1980's: Generating a Scientific Basis for Nursing Practice.
American Nurses Association
Publication No. D-68

Statement on Graduate Education in Nursing.
American Nurses Association
Publication No. NE-5

Statement on Flexible Patterns of Nursing Education.
American Nurses Association
Publication No. NE-3

"The Nursing Market: Where the Jobs Are." *Nursing Opportunities 1982.* Oradell, NJ: Medical Economics Company, 1982.

Westcot, L. "Nursing Education and Nursing Service: A Collaborative Model." *Nursing and Health Care* 2:376, 1981.

APPENDIX I.

Regional and State Offices of the National League for Nursing and the American Nurses Association

---

National League for Nursing

Regional Offices

Midland Region—NLN
111 North Wabash
Suite 1612
Chicago, IL 60602

Northeast Region—NLN
10 Columbus Circle
New York, NY 10019

Southern Region—NLN
50 Executive Park South, N.E.
Atlanta, GA 30329

Western Region—NLN
881 Sneath Lane, Suite 112
P.O. Box 1085
San Bruno, CA 94066

American Nurses Association

State Offices

Alabama State Nurses Association
360 North Hull Street
Montgomery, AL 36197

Alaska Nurses Association
237 East Third Avenue
Anchorage, AK 99501

Arizona Nurses Association
4525 North 12th Street
Phoenix, AZ 85014

Arkansas State Nurses Association
117 South Cedar
Little Rock, AR 72205

California Nurses Association
1855 Folsom Street
Room 670
San Francisco, CA 94103

Colorado Nurses Association
5453 East Evans Place
Denver, CO 80222

Connecticut Nurses Association
One Prestige Drive
Meriden, CT 06450

Delaware Nurses Association
1003 Delaware Avenue, Room 301
Wilmington, DE 19806

District of Columbia Nurses Association
3000 Connecticut Avenue, N.W.
Washington, DC 20008

Florida Nurses Association
Box 6985
Orlando, FL 32853

Georgia Nurses Association
1362 West Peachtree Street, N.W.
Atlanta, GA 30309

Guam Nurses Association
Box 3134
Agana, GU 96910

Hawaii Nurses Association
677 Ala Moana, #1014
Honolulu, HI 96813

Idaho Nurses Association
1134 North Orchard, #8
Boise, ID 83706

Illinois Nurses Association
6 North Michigan Avenue
Chicago, IL 60602

Indiana State Nurses Association
2915 North High School Road
Indianapolis, IN 46224

Appendix I.

Iowa Nurses Association
215 Shops Building
Des Moines, IA 50309

Kansas State Nurses Associatiion
820 Quincy Street, Room 520
Topeka, KS 66612

Kentucky Nurses Association
P.O. Box 8342, Station E
1400 South First Street
St. Louisville, KY 40208

Louisiana State Nurses Association
P.O. Box 837
Metairie, LA 70004

Maine State Nurses Association
62 State Street
P.O. Box 507
Augusta, ME 04330

Maryland Nurses Association
5820 Southwestern Boulevard
Baltimore, MD 21227

Massachusetts Nurses Association
376 Boylston Street
Boston, MA 02116

Michigan Nurses Association
120 Spartan Avenue
East Lansing, MI 48823

Minnesota Nurses Association
1821 University Avenue, Room N-377
St. Paul, MN 55104

Mississippi Nurses Association
135 Bounds Street, Suite 100
Jackson, MS 39206

Missouri Nurses Association
206 East Dunklin Street
P.O. Box 325
Jefferson City, MO 65102

Montana Nurses Association
2001 Eleventh Avenue
P.O. Box 5718
Helena, MT 59604

Nebraska Nurses Association
10730 Pacific Street, Suite 26
Omaha, NE 68114

Nevada Nurses Association
3660 Baker Lane
Reno, NV 89509

New Hampshire Nurses Association
48 West Street
Concord, NH 03301

New Jersey State Nurses Association
320 West State Street
Trenton, NJ 08618

New Mexico Nurses Association
303 Washington, S.E.
Albuquerque, NM 87108

New York State Nurses Association
2113 Western Avenue
Guilderland, NY 12084

162   New Careers in Nursing

North Carolina Nurses Association
Box 12025
Raleigh, NC 27605

North Dakota State Nurses Association
103 1/2 South Third Street
Bismarck, ND 58501

Ohio Nurses Association
4000 East Main Street
P.O. Box 13169
Columbus, OH 43213

Oklahoma Nurses Association
2912 Paseo
Oklahoma City, OK 73103

Oregon Nurses Association
9730 S.W. Cascade Boulevard, Suite 103
Tigard, OR 97223

Pennsylvania Nurses Association
251 North Front Street
Harrisburg, PA 17110

Rhode Island State Nurses Association
H.C. Hall Building (South)
345 Blackstone Boulevard
Providence, RI 02906

South Carolina Nurses Association
1821 Gadsden Street
Columbia, SC 29201

South Dakota Nurses Association
1505 South Minnesota, Suite Six
Sioux Falls, SD 57105

Tennessee Nurses Association
1720 West End Building, Suite 400
Nashville, TN 37203

Texas Nurses Association
314 Highland Mall Boulevard, Suite 504
Austin, TX 78752

Utah Nurse's Association
1058 East Ninth, South
Salt Lake City, UT 84105

Vermont State Nurses Association
72 Hungerford Terrace
Burlington, VT 05401

Virgin Island Nurses Association
P.O. Box 2866
Charlotte Amalie, St. Thomas, VI 00801

Virginia Nurses Association
1311 High Point Avenue
Richmond, VA 23230

Washington State Nurses Association
Fourth and Vine Building, Suite 380
2615 Fourth Avenue
Seattle, WA 98121

West Virginia Nurses Association
Union Building
723 Kanawha Boulevard East, Suite 511
Charleston, WV 25301

Wisconsin Nurses Association
206 East Olin Avenue
Madison, WI 53713

Wyoming Nurses Association
Majestic Building, Room 305
1603 Capitol Avenue
Cheyenne, WY 82001

APPENDIX II.

State Boards of Nursing

ALABAMA

Board of Nursing
State of Alabama
500 East Boulevard, Suite 203
Montgomery, AL 36117

ALASKA

Alaska Board of Nursing
142 East Third Avenue
Anchorage, AK 99501

AMERICAN SAMOA

Health Services Regulatory Board
LBJ Tropical Medical Center
Pago Pago, American Samoa 96799

ARIZONA

Arizona State Board of Nursing
1645 West Jefferson Street, Room 254
Phoenix, AZ 85007

ARKANSAS

Arkansas State Board of Nursing
4120 West Markham
Little Rock, AR 77205

CALIFORNIA

Registered Nursing
1020 North Street
Sacramento, CA 95814

COLORADO

Board of Nursing
1575 Sherman Street, Room 132
Denver, CO 80203

CONNECTICUT

Board of Examiners for Nursing
79 Elm Street, Room 101
Hartford, CT 06115

DELAWARE

Delaware Board of Nursing
Margaret O'Neil Building
Federal and Court Streets
Dover, DE 19901

DISTRICT OF COLUMBIA

District of Columbia
Board of Nursing
614 H Street, Room 112
Washington, DC 20001

FLORIDA

Florida State Board of Nursing
111 East Coastline Drive
Jacksonville, FL 32202

GEORGIA

Board of Examiners for Nurses
166 Pryor Street, S.W.
Atlanta, GA 30303

GUAM

Guam Board of Nurse Examiners
Box 2950
Agana, Guam 96910

HAWAII

Hawaii Board of Nursing
P.O. Box 3469
Honolulu, HI 96801

IDAHO

Idaho State Board of Nursing
Hall of Mirrors
700 West State
Boise, ID 83702

ILLINOIS

Department of Registration and
    Education
55 East Jackson Boulevard
Chicago, IL 60604

Department of Registration and
    Education
320 West Washington Street
Springfield, IL 62786

INDIANA

State Board of Nurses Registration
    and Nursing Education
700 North High School Road, Suite 127
Indianapolis, IN 46224

IOWA

Iowa Board of Nursing
1223 East Court
Des Moines, IA 50319

KANSAS

Kansas State Board of Nursing
503 Kansas Avenue
P.O. Box 1098
Topeka, KS 66601

Appendix II. 165

KENTUCKY

Kentucky Board of Nursing
4010 DuPont Circle
Louisville, KY 40207

LOUISIANA

Louisiana State Board of Nursing
1408 Pere Marquette Building
150 Baronne Street
New Orleans, LA 70112

MAINE

Maine State Board of Nursing
295 Water Street
Augusta, ME 04330

MARYLAND

State Board of Nurse Examiners
State Office Building
201 West Preston Street
Baltimore, MD 21201

MASSACHUSETTS

Board of Nursing Registration
100 Cambridge Street, Room 1509
Boston, MA 02202

MICHIGAN

Michigan Board of Nursing
905 Southland
P.O. Box 30018
Lansing, MI 48909

MINNESOTA

Minnesota Board of Nursing
717 Delaware Street, S.E.
Minneapolis, MN 55414

MISSISSIPPI

Board of Nursing
135 Bounds Street, Suite 101
Jackson, MS 39206

MISSOURI

Missouri State Board of Nursing
3523 North Ten Mile Drive
P.O. Box 656
Jefferson City, MO 65102

MONTANA

Montana State Board of Nursing
Department of Commerce
1424 Ninth Avenue
Helena, MT 59620

NEBRASKA

State Board of Nursing
State House Station, Box 95065
Lincoln, NE 68509

NEVADA

Nevada State Board of Nursing
1135 Terminal Way, Room 209
Reno, NV 89402

NEW HAMPSHIRE

State Board of Nursing
105 Loudon Road
Concord, NH 03301

NEW JERSEY

New Jersey Board of Nursing
1100 Raymond Boulevard, Room 319
Newark, NJ 07102

NEW MEXICO

New Mexico Board of Nursing
5301 Central N.E., Suite 1715
Albuquerque, NM 87108

NEW YORK

New York State Board of Nursing
Office of Professional Education
State Educational Department
Albany, NY 12230

NORTH CAROLINA

North Carolina Board of Nursing
P.O. Box 2129
Raleigh, NC 27602

NORTH DAKOTA

North Dakota Board of Nursing
418 East Rosser Avenue
Bismarck, ND 58505

OHIO

Ohio State Board of Nursing Education
and Nurse Registration
65 South Front Street, Suite 509
Columbus, OH 43215

OKLAHOMA

Oklahoma Board of Nurse Registration
and Nursing Education
4001 North Lincoln, Suite 400
Oklahoma City, OK 73105

OREGON

Oregon State Board of Nursing
1400 S.W. Fifth Avenue, Room 904
Portland, OR 97201

PENNSYLVANIA

Pennsylvania State Board of Nursing
Box 2649
Harrisburg, PA 17105

PUERTO RICO

Puerto Rico Board of Nurse Examiners
800 Roberto H. Todd Avenue
Stop 18
Santurce, PR

RHODE ISLAND

Rhode Island Board of Nursing
Cannon Health Building
75 Davis Street
Providence, RI 02908

SOUTH CAROLINA

South Carolina State Board of Nursing
1777 St. Julian Place, Suite 102
Columbia, SC 29204

SOUTH DAKOTA

South Dakota Board of Nursing
304 South Phillips Avenue, Suite 205
Sioux Falls, SD 57102

TENNESSEE

Tennessee Board of Nursing
TDPH State Office Building
Ben Allen Road
Nashville, TN 37216

TEXAS

Texas Board of Nurse Examiners
510 South Congress, Suite 216
Austin, TX 78704

UTAH

Utah State Board of Nursing
State Office Building, Room 508
Salt Lake City, UT 84111

VERMONT

Vermont Board of Nursing
Pavilion Office Building
109 State Street
Montpelier, VT 05602

VIRGIN ISLANDS

Virgin Islands Board of Nurse Examiners
7309 Charlotte Amalie
St. Thomas, VI 00801

VIRGINIA

Virginia State Board of Nursing
3600 West Broad Street
Richmond, VA 23230

WASHINGTON

Washington State Board of Nursing
Division of Professional Licensing
Box 9649
Olympia, WA 98504

WEST VIRGINIA

West Virginia State Board of Examiners
922 Quarrier Street, Suite 309
Charleston, WV 25301

WISCONSIN

Wisconsin State Division of Nurses
1400 East Washington Avenue, Room 174
Madison, WI 53702

WYOMING

State of Wyoming Board of Nursing
2223 Warren Avenue, Suite One
Cheyenne, WY 82002

APPENDIX III.

Nursing Journals and Publications

AACH

The journal of the Association for the Care of Children in Hospitals.

AANA Journal

The journal of the American Association of Nurse Anesthetists. Serves as an information source for persons interested in anesthesia and the role and functions of the nurse anesthetist.

AANNT Journal

The journal of the American Association of Nephrology Nurses and Technicians. Offers current discussions on direct nursing care, progress and research in nephrology and hemodialysis.

Advances in Nursing Science

The general purpose of this periodical is to share the creative efforts of nurses involved in nursing science. Selections include theory construction, reports on recent research, methodological and ethical issues in nursing research, and issues in nursing education and practice.

American Journal of Nursing (AJN)

The professional journal of the American Nurses Association. Content consists largely of clinical material that enables nurses to keep up-to-date in general nursing practice or to obtain the more detailed information required for specialized practice. It emphasizes content that can be applied in all areas of nursing and presents developments within the profession and the health field at large.

American Journal of Public Health

As the American Public Health Association's official periodical, this journal publishes notes of the annual meeting, announcements of the association and reports of timely research in the field of public health education, assessment and planning.

The American Nurse

The official newspaper of the American Nurses Association. It reports on a broad range of professional, economic, political, ethical and legal issues, and events that affect nursing.

AORN Journal

The Journal of the Association of Operating Room Nurses. Offers nurses original information on nursing practice, administration and issues in operating room nursing. Presents reports from the yearly AORN Congress, regional conferences and selected professional organizations and meetings.

ARN Journal

The journal of the Association of Rehabilitation Nurses. Offers research, discussions and practice "how-to" articles on the art and science of rehabilitation nursing.

Cancer Nursing

Offers contributions of health care professionals involved in the care and prevention of cancer throughout the world. Selections include research reports, discussions on problems and unresolved issues in cancer nursing and important advances in methods of treatment.

Cardiovascular Nursing

A short publication of the American Heart Association that reports current research, trends and practical descriptions of teaching projects and tools that are important for nurses in these specialties.

CCQ: Critical Care Quarterly

Focuses on topics of interest to staff nurses, head nurses and staff development educators in critical care units—coronary and intensive care units as well as emergency departments.

Geriatric Nursing

The journal is for all health professionals providing care to the aged. The editorial content focuses on promoting the well being of the elderly and advanced concepts and practice in the clinical care of the elderly client.

Heart and Lung

An official publication of the American Association of Critical-Care Nurses. Provides discussions on the nursing care of critically ill patients, as well as reports of developments in the field and pertinent research.

Hospitals, J.A.H.A.

The purpose of this journal is to provide current information on developments, issues and important studies in the health care industry.

Image

The formal periodical of Sigma Theta Tau, the nursing honorary society that is dedicated to fostering inquiry, scholarship and leadership in nursing. Pertinent selections include reports of research with important implications for nursing education, practice or administration, as well as views on ethical issues and essays on the function of scientific inquiry in nursing.

Imprint

The magazine of the National Student Nurses Association. The magazine's focus is to serve as a forum on issues facing nursing and society.

Issues in Comprehensive Pediatric Nursing

Discussions outline important everyday nursing procedures and care precautions along with updates on interdisciplinary developments affecting the nursing care of children. Appropriate for nurses involved in pediatrics in both inpatient and outpatient settings, as well as in community health facilities.

Journal of Advanced Nursing

Publishes reports of research and literature reviews on all aspects of professional nursing—practice, research, education and administration. Contains sections on news and book reviews that announce meetings, conferences and resources in England, Ireland, Australia and the United States.

Journal of Continuing Education in Nursing

Currently presents the largest regular selection of research articles related to nursing inservice and continuing education in the United States.

JEN: Journal of Emergency Nursing

Mainly devoted to reports of timely studies on the effective management, process, and practice of teaching nursing in diploma programs, associate degree programs and baccalaureate programs.

Journal of Gerontological Nursing

The purpose of this journal is to provide a forum for sharing information and research, and for scholarly debate on topics pertinent to gerontological nursing or nursing of the elderly.

Journal of Neurosurgical Nursing

The official publication of the American Association of Neurosurgical Nurses. It offers a wide array of useful articles and reports on association meetings and conferences for nurses caring for neurosurgical patients.

Journal of Nurse-Midwifery

A publication of the American College of Nurse-Midwives that focuses on views, experiences, issues and research related to the practice and education of nurse-midwives.

Journal of Nursing Administration (JONA)

Offers selections on research, trends and practices relevant to the functions and tasks of nursing administrators and managers in acute care, long term and community health settings.

Journal of Nursing Care

The official monthly publication of the National Federation of Licensed Practical Nurses. The journal contains articles on new clinical techniques, current developments in all areas of health care, news of legislation and economic security issues, and the activities of the NFLPN.

Journal of Nursing Education

Specializes in research, teaching practices, problems, trends and policy concerns in associate degree, baccalaureate degree and diploma nursing education programs.

JOGN Nursing

(Journal of Obstetric, Gynecologic and Neonatal Nursing). The official publication of the Nurses Association of the American College of Obstetricians and Gynecologists. The purpose of the periodical is to exchange ideas, trends, research, and ethical and policy concerns with those interested in obstetric, gynecologic and neonatal nursing.

Journal of Practical Nursing

The official publication of the National Association for Practical Nurse Education and Service. Contains articles on clinical practice, the role of the practical nurse, and educational issues.

Journal of Psychiatric Nursing and Mental Health Services

Reports of research and creative clinical and educational projects as well as clarifications of complex psychological processes in psychiatric and mental health nursing in acute care and outpatient settings.

MCN

The American Journal of Maternal-Child Nursing. Offers original articles by authorities on their specialties within maternal child nursing. Content includes new material related to clinical practice, articles designed to resensitize nurses in their maternal child nursing practice and issues that professionals should understand to competently function in this field.

Nurse Educator

Presents research, narrative, personal opinion and "how-to" articles on pragmatic and conceptual aspects of nursing education. Content is evenly balanced between staff development education, continuing education and collegiate nursing education.

Nurse Practitioner

The magazine is for those nurses in advanced clinical practice and contains articles on clinical practice and professional issues.

Nursing 82

Offers quick, easy-to-read selections on clinical, educational and employment concerns of practicing nurses in acute care settings.

Nursing Administration Quarterly

Concentrates on the information needs of nursing service administrators and middle managers in acute care and ambulatory care settings.

Nursing and Health Care

The official publication of the National League for Nursing. Content includes articles of clinical, educational, research and political concern.

Nursing Clinics of North America

Issues in this hardbound periodical are devoted to one or two topics of interest to nurses in clinical, educational, administrative and research roles. Includes a variety of theoretical and applied discussions along with reports of relevant research.

Nursing Forum

Contains essays, personal opinion articles and debates on topics of interest to the general nursing audience.

Nursing Leadership

Emphasizes research, discussions and debates on issues related to leadership for nursing practitioners, educators and administrators. Discussions, research articles, "how-to" and personal opinion articles on problems and dilemmas related to leadership roles, decision-making, planning and other leadership activities.

Nursing Management

Contains easy-to-read articles of practical importance to nursing managers, administrators and educators in acute care settings.

Nursing Outlook

Emphasizes current concepts, trends and issues in the nursing profession, especially in relation to nursing education and practice, nursing service administration, community health and health care delivery. It is directed toward nurses who are concerned with those topics and toward other health professionals and lay-persons with a broad interest in nursing and health care matters.

Nursing Research

The journal carries reports, articles, abstracts and other materials to inform members of nursing and other professions of the results of scientific studies in nursing, and to stimulate research in nursing.

Occupational Health Nursing

An official periodical of the American Association of Occupational Health Nurses that focuses on the development and implementation of programs in occupation health units.

Pediatric Nursing

The official periodical of the National Association of Pediatric Nurse Associates and Practitioners. Articles cover a wide spectrum of topics in pediatric nursing—direct care practices and procedures, nursing process concerns, related pharmacology, and growth and development in children—along with discussions of practical interest to nurses in practitioner roles.

Perspectives in Psychiatric Care

Publishes discussions of research, experiences and practices along with interesting debates on issues and developments in psychiatric nursing. Readings focus on both the client and the care-giver and represent a variety of psychological approaches.

Research in Nursing and Health

Reports research by nurses and other health care professionals on relevant topics in nursing and health care. Book reviews and editorials are periodic journal departments. Headings are relevant to the professional learning needs of clinicians, educators and administrators, as well as to researchers.

RN

Provides updates and reviews important day-to-day nursing procedures, national trends and issues pertinent to nurses and nursing assistants who give direct patient care.

Topics in Clinical Nursing

Purpose is to provide helpful resources for nursing clincians who want to deliver total nursing care in health care settings that are frequently fragmented and uncoordinated. Each issue follows one theme, such as "Stress Management."

Western Journal of Nursing Research

This latest research journal focuses on the dissemination of research and research-related material, research reports, essays, book reviews, conferences and meetings, as well as grant announcements, competitions, and regular bylines on research methodology. Intended for nurses in academia, practice and research settings.

Index

Advanced degree programs, 8–11
Adult nurse clinician, 66, 68–69
Air Force Nurse Corp, 121–122, 124, 125
Air Force scholarships, 13–14
Alcohol, Drug Abuse, and Mental Health Administration, 113, 114
American Journal of Nursing (AJN), 1, 168–169
American Nurses Association (ANA), 3, 12, 14, 15, 16, 81
    state offices of, 160–162
Armed Services, 13–14, 112, 121–126
Army Nurse Corp, 121, 122–124, 125
Army scholarships, 13
Army school nurse, 126
Assistant director of nursing, 60–62
Associate degree nursing educator, 138–139
Associate degree programs, 5–6

Baccalaureate degree nursing education, 140–143
Baccalaureate degree programs, 6–8
Burn units, 44

Camp nursing, 87–91
Candy stripers, 15
Center for Disease Control (CDC), 113, 114
Certified nurse midwife, 66, 67, 70–72
Certified registered nurse anesthetist (CRNA), 66, 76–77
Chief nurse executive, 62–63
Civil Service, 112, 126–127
Clinical specialist, 52–56
Clinical specialties, 9–10
College health service, nurse practitioner, 77–79
Collegiate nursing programs, 138
Combined careers, 152–156
    combined teaching and practice positions, 155–156
    international consultation, 154–155
    nurse editor, 153–154
    nursing school recruiter, 155

Commissioned Officer Student Training Program (COSTP), 114
Community health nursing, 10, 81–84, 97–99
    camp, 87–91
    occupational health, 92–97
    rural, 91–92
    schools, 66, 77–79, 85–87
Cumulative Index to Nursing and Allied Health Literature, 12

Day surgery unit, 26–27
Degrees, nursing
    associate, 5–6
    baccalaureate, 6–8
    doctoral, 10–11
    master's, 8–10
Detoxification units, 47
Developmentally disabled children, nursing, 106–107
Diploma nursing education, 4, 136–137
Diploma programs, 4
Director of nursing, 62–63
Doctoral degree nursing education, 144–146
Doctoral degree nursing programs, 10–11

Editor, nurse, 153–154
Education, 3–18
    advanced degrees, 8–11
    assistant director of nursing, 60–62
    careers in nursing, 134–147
    choosing a nursing program, 11–13
    clinical specialist, 56
    financial aid, 13–14
    for an expanded practice role, 68
    head nurse, 56–58
    Indian Health Service, 115–121
    in-service educator, 49–52
    nurse practitioners and clinicians, 68
    practical nursing programs, 3
    registered nurses, 3–11
    school nurses, 86
Educational administration, 146–147
EENT units, 46

Emergency room nurse practitioner, 66
Emergency room, nursing in, 27–29
Emotionally disturbed children, school nurse for, 86–87
Extended care facilities, 110–111
    developmentally disabled children, nursing for, 106–107
    geriatric nurse practitioner, 101
    gerontological nurse specialist, 102–103
    hospice care, 108–110
    nursing homes, 100–101
    rehabilitation centers, 104–106

Family nurse clinician, 66, 69
Family planning nurse practitioner, 66, 70–71
Food and Drug Administration (FDA), 113, 114
Functional nursing, 49

Geriatric nurse practitioner (GNP), 101
Geriatrics, 9
Gerontological nurse specialist (GNS), 102–103
Government service, 112–133
    Armed Services, 13–14, 112, 121–126
    Civil Service, 112, 126–127
    Indian Health Service, 113, 115–121, 127
    nursing during war, 130–132
    Peace Corps and Vista, 130
    Public Health Service, 112–115, 127
    Veteran's Administration, 127–130
Graduate degree programs, 8–9
Gynecological units, 46

Head nurse, 56–60
Health maintenance organizations (HMOs), 82
Health Resources Administration, 115
Health Services Administration, 115
Hospice care, 108–110
Hospitals, nursing in, 19, 63–65
    assistant director, 60–62
    chief nurse executive, 62–63
    clinical specialist, 52–56
    director of nursing, 62–63
    functional nursing, 49
    head nurse, 56–60
    in-service educator, 49–52
    job hierarchies, 59
    primary nursing, 48
    staff nursing, 20–47
    team nursing, 48–49

Independent practices, 66–68, 79–80
    certified registered nurse anesthetist, 76–77
    college health service, 77–79
    neonatal nurse practitioner, 66, 75–76
    psychiatric nurse practitioner, 74–75
Indian Health Service (INS), 113, 115–118, 127
    locations for nursing positions, 118–121
Infection control, 44
In-service educator, 49–52
Intensive care unit (ICU), 9, 44–45
    newborn, 37–39
    surgical, 29–32
International consultation, 154–155

Job hierarchies, hospitals, 59
Joint practices, 66–68, 79–80
    adult nurse clinician, 66, 68–69
    certified nurse midwife, 66, 67, 70–72
    family nurse clinician, 66, 69
    pediatric nurse clinician, 66, 73–74
Journals and publications, nursing, 168–176

Labor and delivery unit, 34–37
License, obtaining RN, 3
Licensed practical nurses (LPNs), 3, 20, 48
Loans, student, 14

Master's degree nursing education, 143–144
Master's degree programs, 8–10
Medical-surgical nursing, 9
Medical units, 45
Midwifery, 9, 66, 67, 70–72

National Health Service Corps, 113
National Institutes of Health (NIH), 113, 115
National League for Nursing (NLN), 4, 11, 14, 15, 16
    regional and state offices of, 159
Native americans, 113, 115–121
Navy Nurse Corp, 121–122, 123, 124–125
Neonatal nurse practitioner, 75–76
Neurology, 9
Neurosurgery, 22–26
Newborn intensive care unit (NICO), 37–39
Newborn transport nursing, 39–40
Nurse editor, 153–154

Index 179

Nurse educators
    Associate degree nursing education, 138–139
    baccalaureate degree nursing education, 140–143
    collegiate programs, 138
    diploma nursing education, 4, 136–137
    doctoral degree nursing education, 144–146
    educational administration, 146–147
    master's degree nursing education, 143–144
    practical nursing education, 143–144
Nurse practitioners and clinicians, 79–80
    adult, 66, 68–69
    certified nurse anesthetist, 66, 76–77
    certified nurse midwife, 66, 70–72
    college health service, 77–79
    emergency room, 66
    family, 66, 69
    family planning, 66, 70–71
    geriatric, 101
    gerontologic, 66
    neonatal, 66, 75–76
    obstetric and gynecologic, 66
    pediatric, 66, 73–74
    psychiatric, 66, 74–75
    school, 10, 66, 77–79
Nursing, 1–3, 156–158
    assistant director of, 60–62
    careers in education, 134–147
    combined careers, 152–156
    community health, 81–99
    director of, 62–63
    educational programs for practical, 3
    educational programs for registered nurses, 3–9, 10–18
    independent and joint practices, 66–80
    in extended care facilities, 100–111
    in government service, 112–133
    in hospitals, 19–65
    journals and publications, 168–176
    research, 147–152
    state boards of, 163–167
Nursing school recruiter, 155
Nursing homes, 100–101

Obstetrics and gynecology, 9, 34–37, 46, 66
Occupational health nursing, 92–97
Oncology units, 47
Operating room, 22–27
Orthopedic units, 46
Outpatient clinic, 40–43

Peace Corps, 1, 112, 130
Pediatric nurse clinician, 66, 73–74
Pediatric units, 9, 44
Practical nursing education, 134–136
Practical nursing programs, 3
Practice positions, 155–156
Primary care nursing, 10, 48
Private duty nursing, 47
Psychiatric-mental health nursing, 10
Psychiatric nurse practitioner, 74–75
Psychiatric unit, nursing in, 32–34
Public Health Service, 112–114
    health agencies of, 114–115

Recruiter, nursing school, 155
Registered nurses (RNs), 3–19, 48
Rehabilitation centers, 104–106
Research, 46, 147–152
Research units, 46
RN license, obtaining, 3
Rural nursing, 91–92

Scholarships, 13–14
School nursing, 10, 66, 77–79, 85–86
    Army, 126
    emotionally disturbed children, 86–87
Specialist, clinical, 52–56
Specialties, clinical, 9–10
Staff nursing, 20, 43
    burn units, 44
    detoxification units, 47
    EENT units, 46
    emergency room, 27–29
    gynecological units, 46
    infection control, 44
    intensive care units, 9, 44–45
    labor and delivery units, 34–37
    medical units, 45
    newborn intensive care unit, 37–39
    newborn transport nursing, 39–40
    oncology units, 47
    operating room, 22–27
    orthopedic units, 46
    outpatient clinic, 40–43
    pediatric units, 44

    private duty nursing, 47
    psychiatric unit, 32–34
    research units, 46
    surgical intensive care unit, 29–32
    surgical unit, 20–22
    temporary agency nursing, 47
    transplant units, 46–47
State boards of nursing, 163–167
Student loans, 14
Surgical intensive care unit, 29–32
Surgical unit, 20–22
    day surgery unit, 26–27

Teaching, careers in, 134–147
    combined teaching, 155–156
Team nursing, 48–49
Temporary agency nursing, 47
Transplant units, 46–47

Veteran's Administration (VA), 127–130
Vista, 112, 130
Volunteer work, 15

War, nursing during, 130–132
Work-study programs, 14